For nurse	For nurse educator	For nurse administrator
• The blood bag details (Patient name, UHID, blood group, Expiry date) must be checked.	• Train nurses on Blood Transfusion SOP. • Reiterate on Patient identification.	• Create a robust policy for blood transfusion involving blood bank, Nursing and medical

Learning Aspects from the respective events for nurses, educators and administrators have been dealt with separately for delivering better clinical services.

E—Learning Ignited from Errors (A Handbook on Patient Safety Events)

O did not cross check the blood bag with the patient's file for the od group report

rse failed to reconfirm the patient's blood group just before starting blood transfusion in the presence of another senior nurse.

was a total breakdown in following safe blood transfusion protocols.

ons Learned

nurse	For nurse educator	For nurse administrator
he blood bag details Patient name, UHID, blood group, Expiry date) must be checked. These identifiers must be matched with the same information in the patient's file and cross-matched report and patient identification band.	• Train nurses on Blood Transfusion SOP. • Reiterate on Patient identification. • Include blood transfusion policy in nurse's induction training. • Assess training needs based on audits and incidents reported and facilitate training as required.	• Create a robust policy for blood transfusion involving blood bank, Nursing and medical departments • Conduct root cause analysis and corrective and preventive actions (CAPA) for such incidents.

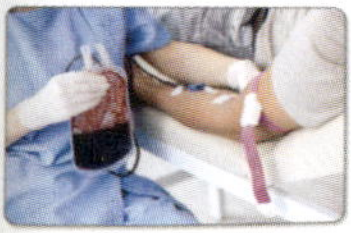

Figure 11 Blood transfusion stopped immediately

vent-Based Learning Summary

the realm of patient care, it is imperative that nurses prioritize patient safety, pecially during blood transfusions. Always double-check patient details such names, and UHID to ensure they match the ID band, blood form, label on the ood bag.

AF520539

5 **Event-Based Learning Summary**

In the realm of patient care, it is imperative that nurses prioritize patient safety, especially during blood transfusions. Always double-check patient details such as names, and UHID to ensure they match the ID band, blood form, label on the blood bag. Verify the patient's blood group, reconfirm it before the transfusion begins, and include patient identifiers in every step of the process. If any discrepancies arise, take immediate action by stopping the transfusion, notifying the healthcare team, and following their guidance. Effective communication within the healthcare team is vital for error prevention and swift resolution. These precautions and commitment to patient safety are essential to prevent identification errors and ensure that the right blood products are administered to the right patients, ultimately saving lives and upholding the highest standard of care.

Each event ends with the **Event-Based Learning Summary** segment, that sets you to wrap the learnings as take away to make your practice safer and keep your patients well-protected.

ASSOCIATION OF NURSE EXECUTIVES (INDIA)
PASSION TO ACTION

Association of Nurse Executives (India)

LIFE

Learning Ignited from Errors

(A Handbook on Patient Safety Events)

Editors

Thankam Gomez RN, RM, BSN (UCOL, NZ)
Founder CEO
Cygnia Healthcare, Gurugram
Past President & Founder Member – ANEI

Jaideep Herbert RN, RM, MSN, PhD
Chief Operating Officer
Vidyanta Medical Simulation Center, Gurugram
Member – ANEI

Foreword

Capt. Ajitha Nair
Managing Director
HealBiz, Kerala
National President
Association of Nurse Executives (India)

CBSPD
Dedicated to Education

CBS Publishers & Distributors Pvt Ltd

• New Delhi • Bengaluru • Chennai • Kochi • Kolkata • Lucknow • Mumbai
• Hyderabad • Jharkhand • Nagpur • Patna • Pune • Uttarakhand

DISCLAIMER

All names and characters mentioned in this book are entirely fictional. While the events are based on real-life incidents, any resemblance to actual persons, living or deceased, is purely coincidental.

Association of Nurse Executives (India)

LIFE

Learning Ignited from Errors

(A Handbook on Patient Safety Events)

ISBN: 978-93-94525-43-6

First Edition: 2025

Published by **Satish Kumar Jain** and produced by **Varun Jain** for

CBS Publishers and Distributors Pvt Ltd

4819/XI Prahlad Street, 24 Ansari Road, Daryaganj, New Delhi 110 002, India.

Ph: +91-11-23289259, 23266861, 23266867 Website: www.cbspd.com

Fax: 011-23243014

e-mail: delhi@cbspd.com; cbspubs@airtelmail.in.

Corporate Office: 204 FIE, Industrial Area, Patparganj, Delhi 110 092

Ph: +91-11-4934 4934 Fax: 4934 4935

e-mail: feedback@cbspd.com; bhupesharora@cbspd.com

Branches

- **Bengaluru:** Seema House 2975, 17th Cross, K.R. Road, Banasankari 2nd Stage, Bengaluru-560 070, Karnataka
  Ph: +91-80-26771678/79 Fax: +91-80-26771680 e-mail: bangalore@cbspd.com
- **Chennai:** 7, Subbaraya Street, Shenoy Nagar, Chennai-600 030, Tamil Nadu
  Ph: +91-44-26680620, 26681266 Fax: +91-44-42032115 e-mail: chennai@cbspd.com
- **Kochi:** 68/1534, 35, 36-Power House Road, Opp. KSEB, Cochin-682018, Kochi, Kerala
  Ph: +91-484-4059061-65 Fax: +91-484-4059065 e-mail: kochi@cbspd.com
- **Kolkata:** Hind Ceramics Compound, 1st Floor, 147, Nilganj Road, Belghoria, Kolkata-700056, West Bengal
  Ph: +033-2563-3055/56 e-mail: kolkata@cbspd.com
- **Lucknow:** Basement, Khushnuma Complex, 7-Meerabai Marg (Behind Jawahar Bhawan), Lucknow-226001, Uttar Pradesh
  Ph: +0522-4000032 e-mail: tiwari.lucknow@cbspd.com
- **Mumbai:** PWD Shed, Gala No. 25/26, Ramchandra Bhatt Marg, Next to J.J. Hospital Gate No. 2, Opp. Union Bank of India, Noor Baug, Mumbai-400009, Maharashtra
  Ph: +91-22-66661880/89 Fax: +91-22-24902342 e-mail: mumbai@cbspd.com

Representatives

- **Hyderabad** +91-9885175004
- **Nagpur** +91-9421945513
- **Pune** +91-9623451994
- **Jharkhand** +91-9811541605
- **Patna** +91-9334159340
- **Uttarakhand** +91-9716462459

Printed at: Magic International Pvt. Ltd., Greater Noida, UP, India

CBS Nursing Knowledge Tree

Extends its Tribute to

Florence Nightingale

For glorifying the role of women as nurses,
For holding the title of " The Lady with the Lamp,"
For working tirelessly for humanity–
Florence Nightingale will always be
remembered for her
selfless and memorable services to the
human race.

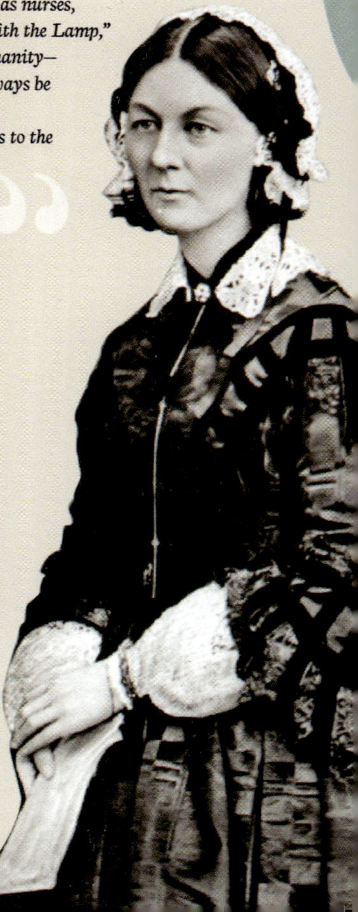

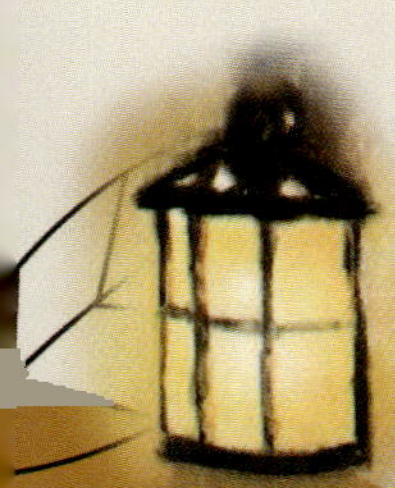

Florence Nightingale
(May 1820 – August 1910)

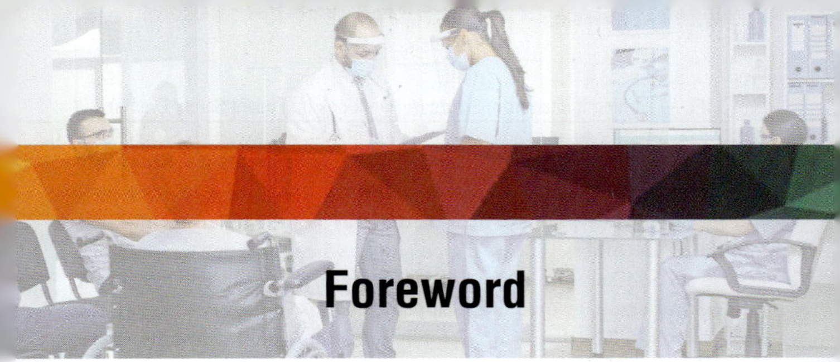

Foreword

We, at the Association of Nurse Executives (India), strive every moment to live up to our motto, Passion to Action. *Learning Ignited from Errors (LIFE)* is yet another testament to the unwavering commitment toward making our workplaces and practices safer for patients and staff. Quality of healthcare undeniably means reliability of what is done in the name of healthcare, i.e., the intent and outcome of our actions are the same. The patient seeks healthcare for managing a health issue, and we plan and act with the same intent and it is achieved during the delivery of healthcare. But the stark reality is destined to be different. Despite our best intent, things go horribly wrong during the process of delivering healthcare in many cases, and the healthcare workers and patients are caught in the midst of adverse outcomes, errors and suffering that result from such events. We talk less or never about it due to fear of judgmental attitude of people around us and the public at large, and continue to suffer in silence. This happens because of the sheer lack of understanding of quality in healthcare as a science in general and the interplay between causative factors behind errors in particular.

In India, there have been minimal or no attempts in talking about the truth related to healthcare errors unlike in the western world. *Learning Ignited from Errors (LIFE)* is a brave attempt of discussing what has gone wrong while providing patient care. It was not an easy task to talk about it again; and while sharing, I am sure the nurses must have lived through the pain of committing an unintended and unwanted error.

This book is a collection of 100 such errors and the lessons learned thereof, offering a profound glimpse into the world of healthcare from the perspective of those who stand at its frontline—the nurses. It is a testament to their courage and resilience, as they openly share their experiences, not to dwell on mistakes but to illuminate the path toward safer practices and better patient outcomes.

I sincerely hope that this book inspires the readers to see errors not as weaknesses but as an opportunity to learn about the science of errors so that each one of us can have warnings just like the roadside signboard: "accident-prone area, drive carefully".

The best way to live our commitment to patients as healthcare workers is by learning from our mistakes and translating this learning into modifying the practice. Yet smarter way is to learn from mistakes committed by others. It can happen only when one musters courage against all odds to speak the truth and the listeners accept it without judging the person. I would like to applaud all those nurses who shared the errors committed by them with us for demonstrating their commitment to saving patients from healthcare-related errors through the lessons learned and adopting safer practices. We have made all the events anonymous in these narrations to safeguard the people and places.

Dr Rosaline Rachel, the Principal of the prestigious and legendary Madras Medical Mission College of Nursing, Chennai, who chairs the Education Committee of the Association of Nurse Executives (India), with her team members, has strived to collect this profound and invaluable resource. As we delve into these stories, we are reminded of the importance of continuously embracing lessons that emerge from errors. Through this shared commitment, we contribute to creating a healthcare landscape that is not only safer but also more compassionate.

May the pages of this book serve as a guiding light toward a future healthcare where patient safety is prioritized by all stakeholders and is defined and delivered by professionals who have the better and right understanding of the nuances of healthcare-related errors, who can error-proof the processes of care delivery and safeguard the interests of patients, staff, and management alike.

I have no doubt that this book has the potential to generate powerful discussions that will foster more learning and pave the way for better patient care in all settings. I would like to thank and congratulate all the contributors, reviewers and editors as well as CBS Publishers and Distributors for undertaking this task.

Capt. Ajitha Nair
Managing Director
HealBiz, Kerala
National President
Association of Nurse Executives (India)

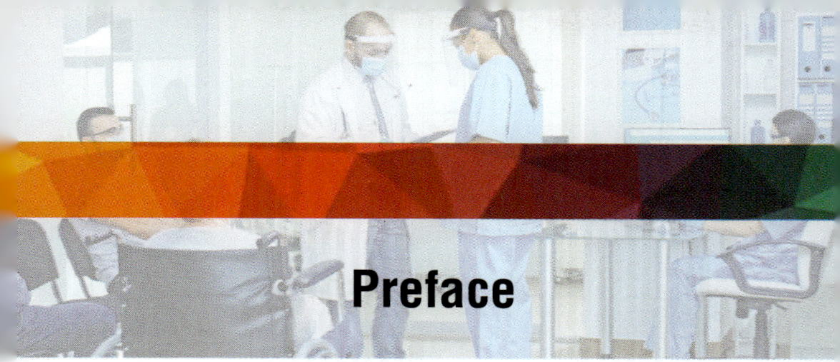

Preface

In the realm of healthcare, every error must serve as a guiding light, leading us toward a future of unwavering patient safety and well-being. *Learning Ignited from Errors (LIFE)* is more than just a book; it stands as a testament to the resilience and unwavering dedication of nurses who tirelessly work to enhance patient care, even in the face of the most formidable challenges.

Contained within these pages is a treasury of 100 real-life accounts of errors experienced by nurses. These stories are not mere accounts of missteps; they represent the profound commitment to learning and growth that defines the nursing profession. As we delve into the intricacies of each error, we unravel the threads of knowledge that pave the way for safer practices and improved outcomes.

The core of this book is an unyielding focus on patient safety. With every error shared, a solution emerges, a lesson is learned, and a solemn promise is made to prevent such misfortunes from recurring. It is a tribute to the nurses who convert setbacks into stepping stones, utilizing their experiences to illuminate a path toward excellence in healthcare.

As you embark on this voyage of learning, do not perceive each error as a blemish but as a spark that kindles the flames of progress. Let these stories spark conversations, cultivate a culture of transparency, and stoke the fire of continuous improvement. Together, we can transform the pages of this book into a testament to our collective dedication to patient safety.

In the spirit of growth and learning, we extend an invitation to join us in embracing the invaluable lessons that arise from errors. By doing so, you contribute to forging a healthcare landscape that is safer, more compassionate, and committed to the well-being of every patient.

Please refer all acronyms before reading the book.

Let the journey begin...

Acknowledgments

In 2017, the Association of Nurse Executives (India) was founded with a resolute commitment to prioritize patient safety at its core. This association of nurse leaders recognizes the paramount importance of working toward "Zero Harm" to patients in healthcare settings. In a world where, as the adage goes, "To Err is Human," this book, titled *Learning Ignited from Errors (LIFE)*, underscores the vital notion that learning from real events and near misses is the most effective way to prevent patient harm.

A team led by Dr Rosaline Rachel and co-chaired by Dr Geeta Parwanda, the Education Committee of the association, along with its dedicated members, embarked on a mission to gather real-life patient safety events from across the nation. The result of their collective efforts is this comprehensive collection of 100 events, with contributions from 41 dedicated individuals. Many of these stories revolve around the International Patient Safety Goals, making them highly relevant to the clinical setting.

One of the distinguishing features of this book is its accessibility. Written in an easy-to-understand language, it ensures quick comprehension, making it an invaluable resource for nurses, nursing students, nurse educators, and nursing administrators alike. Our vision for this book is to become a staple in all nursing schools, colleges, and hospitals committed to enhancing patient safety. After all, we cannot afford to make every mistake to learn from them.

Learning Ignited from Errors (LIFE) is an extraordinary team effort that reflects the unwavering dedication and commitment of the Education Committee and members of the Association of Nurse Executives (India). It serves as a beacon, guiding healthcare professionals toward a future where patient safety is paramount, errors are minimized, and excellence in nursing care prevails.

We invite you to delve into the stories within these pages, to learn, to grow, and to contribute to a healthcare landscape where "Zero Harm" becomes a reality.

We extend our heartfelt gratitude to the esteemed former officials of the association for their approval to embark on this journey. Ms Thankam Gomez (President), Dr Jothi Clara Michael (Vice President), Ms Shubhada Sakurikar (Secretary), and Capt. Ajitha Nair (Treasurer), all have played a pivotal role in making this endeavor possible.

However, this book would not have been evolved into reality without the tireless efforts of the members of the Education Committee. Ms Eshita Chanda, Ms Thankam Gomez, Dr Rebecca Samson, Ms Anisha Vadakkepatt, Dr Bhuneshwari Dash, Dr Jayasankari S, Ms Kripa Angeline A, Ms Suchitra Dalvi, and Ms Vinette Saldanha, who under the able leadership of the Chair and Vice-Chair of the committee have worked relentlessly to collect and compile these invaluable narratives.

We also extend our special gratitude to our dedicated reviewers and editors who, despite their busy schedules, committed themselves wholeheartedly toward shaping this book. Their passion for patient safety has undoubtedly enriched the content and elevated its significance.

As we move forward on this remarkable journey through *Learning Ignited from Errors (LIFE)*, we are reminded of the power of collaboration, dedication, and a shared vision. May this effort reach thousands of nurses, igniting learning and thereby making the hospitals a safer place for patients.

Education Committee
Association of Nurse Executives (India)

Editors and Reviewers

Editors

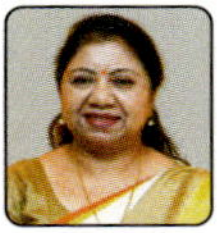

Thankam Gomez
RN, RM, BSN (UCOL.NZ)

Founder CEO
Cygnia Healthcare, Gurugram

Past President &
Founder Member – ANEI

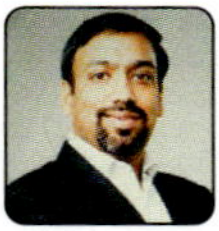

Jaideep Herbert
RN, RM, MSN, PhD

Chief Operating Officer
Vidyanta Medical Simulation Center
Gurugram

Member – ANEI

Reviewers

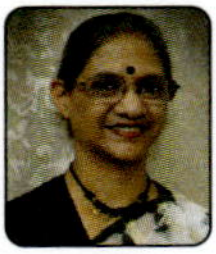

Abanti Gopan
RN, RM, MPhil (N)

Nursing Consultant & Guest Faculty
Freelance for PG Nursing

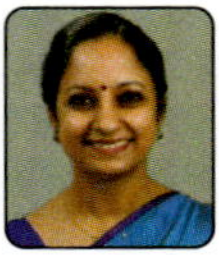

Ajitha Nair
RN, RM, MSN

Managing Director
HealBiz, Kerala

National President &
Founder Member – ANEI

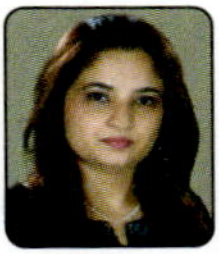

Annu Kaushik
RN, RM, PhD (N)

Director – Nursing
Cloudnine Group of Hospitals

Executive Member – ANEI

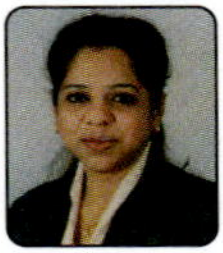

Elizabeth Joseph
RN, RM, MSN, PhD (N)

Chief of Nursing & Quality
Mumbai Central, Mumbai

Founder Member – ANEI

The names of the reviewers are arranged in an alphabetical order.

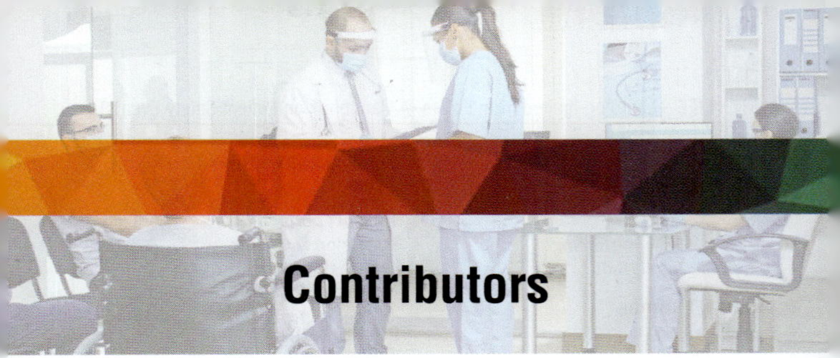

Contributors

Ajee K L
RN, RM, PhD (N)
Professor & HOD
(Foundation of Nursing)
Amrita College of Nursing
Kochi, Kerala

Amita Naze
RN, RM, MBA
Nursing Superintendent
Sree Narayana Institute of
Medical Science
Ernakulam, Kerala

Anisha Vadakkepatt
RN, RM, MSc (N)
Lecturer
Amrita College of Nursing
Kochi, Kerala

Anita Kiruba Jayakumar
RN, RM, MSc (N)
Professor/Nurse Manager
Internal Quality Assurance
Cell Coordinator
College of Nursing
CMC, Vellore, Tamil Nadu

Anusha Anand K
RN, RM
Tutor
MMM College of Nursing
Chennai, Tamil Nadu

Baby Lakshmi
RN, RM, MSc (N)
Deputy Head Nursing Operations
Mehta Multispeciality Hospitals
Chennai, Tamil Nadu

Bijaya Thongam
RN, RM, PhD (N)
Professor
Asian Institute of Nursing Education
Guwahati, Assam

Eshita Chanda
RN, RM, MSc (N)
Assistant General Manager Nursing
Asian Institute of Gastroenterology
Hyderabad, Telangana

Geetha Parwanda
RN, RM, PhD (N)
Principal & Dean
Faculty of Nursing
Subharti University
Meerut, Uttar Pradesh

Himanshi
RN, RM, MSc (N) & MBA
Clinical Coordinator/Assistant Professor
Teerthanker Mahaveer University
Moradabad, Uttar Pradesh

Jaya Shankari S
RN, RM, PhD (N)
Vice Principal
College of Nursing, PIMS
Pondicherry

Leena Chandrasekaran
RN, RM, MSc (N)
Group Head Nursing Operations
Mehta Multispeciality Hospitals
Chennai, Tamil Nadu

The names of the contributors are arranged in an alphabetical order.

Jenilin Sujatha P
RN, RM
Tutor
MMM College of Nursing
Chennai, Tamil Nadu

Julin K Thomas
RN, RM, MSc (N)
Assistant Professor
MMM College of Nursing
Chennai, Tamil Nadu

Kavitha M
RN, RM, PhD (N)
Professor
Meenakshi College of Nursing
Chennai, Tamil Nadu

Kingsle Kishore Coumar M F
RN, RM, PhD (N)
ANS – Quality & Accreditation
Mahatma Gandhi Medical College and Research Institute
Puducherry

Kripa Angeline A
RN, RM, PhD (N)
Professor cum Nursing Superintendent
Mahatma Gandhi Medical College and Research Institute
Puducherry

Krishna Choudhury
RN, RM, MSc (N), PhD Scholar
Associate Professor
NEMCARE Institute of Nursing Sciences
Mirza, Assam

Latha U S
RN, RM, MSc (N), MA (Sociology)
Assistant Professor
M S Ramaiah Institute of Nursing Education and Research
Bengaluru, Karnataka

Mahalakshmi
RN, RM, MSc (N)
Tutor
MMM College of Nursing
Chennai, Tamil Nadu

Priyanka Shirsath
RN, RM, MSc (N)
Clinical Coordinator
Education & Quality
Gleneagles Global Hospital
Mumbai, Maharashtra

Pushpalatha
RN, RM, MSc (N), MBA
Head Nursing Operations
Mehta Multispeciality Hospitals
Chennai, Tamil Nadu

Ramya S N
RN, RM, MSc (N)
Assistant Professor
M S Ramaiah Institute of Nursing Education and Research
Bengaluru, Karnataka

Regina P F
RN, RM, PhD (N)
Associate Professor & HOD (OBG Nursing)
Nehru College of Nursing
Palakkad, Kerala

Rema Muktieh
RN, RM, MSc (N)
Assistant Professor
MMM College of Nursing
Chennai, Tamil Nadu

Rosaline Rachel
RN, RM, PhD (N)
Principal
MMM College of Nursing
Chennai, Tamil Nadu

Roselin Anitha
RN, RM, MSc (N)
Tutor
MMM College of Nursing
Chennai, Tamil Nadu

Rujula Tejkumar Patil
RN, RM
Senior Nursing-Incharge

The names of the contributors are arranged in an alphabetical order.

S Ruth Kezia
RN, RM, MSc (N)
Tutor
MMM College of Nursing
Chennai, Tamil Nadu

Sasikala P
RN, RM, MSc (N)
Tutor
MMM College of Nursing
Chennai, Tamil Nadu

Shini M
RN, RM, MSc (N)
Assistant Professor
MMM College of Nursing
Chennai, Tamil Nadu

Shiny Varghese
RN, RM, MBA (HCS)
Head Nursing
Manipal Hospital Whitefield
Bengaluru, Karnataka

Snehal Suhas Mayekar
RN, RM
Assistant Professor
MMM College of Nursing
Chennai, Tamil Nadu

Sonali Gupta
RN, RM
Senior Staff Nurse
Bhaktivedanta Hospital &
Research Institute
Mumbai, Maharashtra

Soujanya Kesara
RN, RM, MSc (N), PGDHHM
Nursing Manager
Rainbow Hospitals
Nanakramguda, Hyderabad, Telangana

Suja Kumari S
RN, RM, MSc (N)
Assistant Professor
Amrita College of Nursing
Kochi, Kerala

Thankam Gomez
RN, RM, BSN (UCOL, NZ)
Founder CEO
Cygnia Healthcare, Gurugram, Haryana
Past President &
Founder Member – ANEI

Vidhi Ghadi
RN, RM
Head Nurse
Bhaktivedanta Hospital &
Research Institute
Mumbai, Maharashtra

Vinette Saldanha
RN, RM
Chief of Nursing
HCG Cancer Centre
Borivali, Mumbai, Maharashtra

Vinod Kumaar
RN, RM, MSc (N), FECMO
Clinical Specialist
Molnlycke Healthcare
Gurugram, Haryana

Suchitra Sham Dalvi
RN, RM, MSc (N)
Nursing Superintendent
Bhaktivedanta Hospital &
Research Institute
Mumbai, Maharashtra

The names of the contributors are arranged in an alphabetical order.

From the Publisher's Desk

Dear Reader,

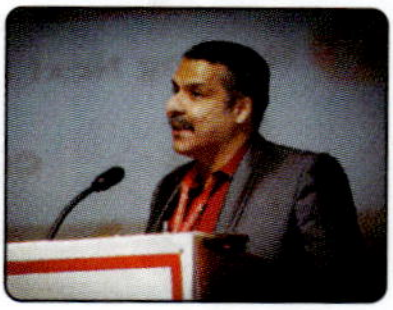

Nursing Education has a rich history, often characterized by traditional teaching techniques that have evolved over time. Primarily, teaching took place within classroom settings. Lectures, textbooks, and clinical rotations were the core teaching tools; and students majorly relied on textbooks by local or foreign publishers for quality education. However, today, technology has completely transformed the field of nursing education, making it an integral part of the curriculum. It has evolved to include a range of technological tools that enhance the learning experience and better prepare students for clinical practice.

As publishers, we've been contributing to the field of Medical Science, Nursing and Allied Sciences and earned the trust of many. By supporting **Indian authors**, coupled with **nursing webinars and conferences**, we have paved an easier path for aspiring nurses, empowering them to excel in national and state level exams. With this, we're not only enhancing the quality of patient care but also enabling future nurses to adapt to new challenges and innovations in the rapidly evolving world of healthcare. Following the ideology of **Bringing learning to people instead of people going for learning**, so far, we've been doing our part by:

- Developing quality content by qualified and well-versed authors
- Building a strong community of faculty and students
- Introducing a smart approach with Digital/Hybrid Books, and
- Offering simulation Nursing Procedures, etc.

Innovative teaching methodologies, such as modern-age Phygital Books, have sparked the interest of the Next-Gen students in pursuing advanced education. The enhancement of educational standards through **Omnipresent Knowledge Sharing Platforms** has further facilitated learning, bridging the gap between doctors and nurses.

At Nursing Next Live, a sister concern of CBS Publishers & Distributors, we have long recognized the immense potential within the nursing field. Our journey in innovating nursing education has allowed us to make substantial and meaningful contributions. With the vision of strengthening learning at every stage, we have introduced several plans that cater to the specific needs of the students, including but not limited to **Plan UG** for undergraduates, **Plan MSc** for postgraduate aspirants, **Plan FDP** for upskilling faculties, **SDL** for integrated learning and **Plan NP** for bridging the gap between theoretical & practical learning. Additionally, we have successfully completed seven series of our **Target High** Book in a very short period, setting a milestone in the education industry. We have been able to achieve all this just with the sole vision of laying the foundation of diversified knowledge for all. With the rise of a new generation of educated, tech-savvy individuals, we anticipate even more remarkable advancements in the coming years.

We take immense pride in our achievements and eagerly look forward to the future, brimming with new opportunities for innovation, growth and collaborations with experienced minds such as yourself who can contribute to our mission as Authors, Reviewers and/or Faculties. Together, let's foster a generation of nurses who are confident, competent, and prepared to succeed in a technology-driven healthcare system.

Mr Bhupesh Aarora

(Sr Vice President – Publishing & Marketing)

bhupeshaarora@cbspd.com| +91 95553 53330

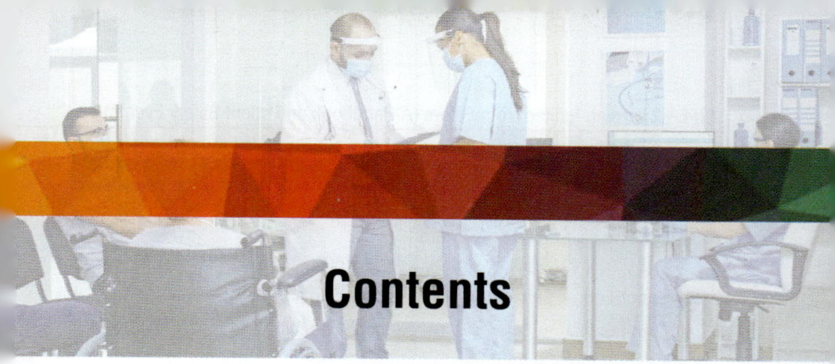

Contents

*PSE, patient safety event

Contd...

Contd...

Contd...

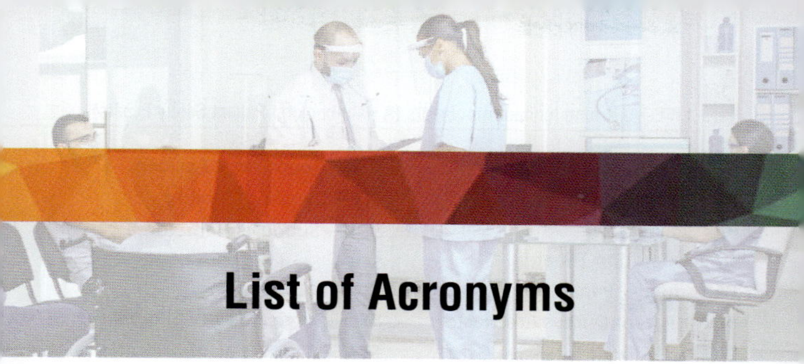

List of Acronyms

ABG – Arterial Blood Gases

ADR – Adverse Drug Reaction

AKI – Acute Kidney Injury

APTT – Activated Partial Thromboplastin Time

BD – "bis in die" meaning twice a day

CAD – Coronary Artery Disease

CAPA – Corrective Preventive Action

CBC – Complete Blood Count

CBG – Capillary Blood Glucose

CCM – Critical Care Medicine

CCU – Coronary Care Unit

CKD – Chronic Kidney Disease

CM – Coming Morning

CS – Cesarean Section

CT – Computed Tomography

CUS – Concerned, Uncomfortable, Safety Issue

CVA – Cerebrovascular Accident

CVC – Central Venous Catheter

DM – Diabetes Mellitus

DVT – Deep Vein Thrombosis

ECG – Electrocardiogram

EMS – Emergency Medical Services

ERCP – Endoscopic Retrograde Cholangiopancreatography

EUS – Endoscopic Ultrasound

FBS – Fasting Blood Sugar

FCM – Ferric Carboxymaltose

FHR – Fetal Heart Rate

GCS – Glasgow Coma Scale

GDA – General Duty Assistant

GDM – Gestational Diabetes Mellitus

HDU – High Dependency Unit

HTN – Hypertension

ICD – Intercostal Drainage

ID – Identification

IPD – In-Patient Department

IPSG – International Patient Safety Goal

IT – Information Technology

IV – Intravenous

LASA – Look Alike Sound Alike

LSCS – Lower Segment Cesarean Section

MAR – Medication Administration Record

MOI – Mechanism of Injury

NICU – Neonatal Intensive Care Unit

NPO – Nil Per Oral

NSI – Needle Stick Injury

NS – Normal Saline

OD – Omne in die or "once daily"

OHAs – Oral Hypoglycemic Agents

OPD – Outpatient Department

ORIF – Open Reduction and Internal Fixation

OT – Operation Theater

PAP smear – Papanicolaou smear

PDA – Patent Ductus Arteriosus

PICU – Pediatric Intensive Care Unit

POD – Post Operative Day

PPC – Puncture Proof Container

PSE – Patient-Safety Event

PTCA – Percutaneous Transluminal Coronary Angioplasty

PUSH – Pressure Ulcer Scale for Healing

RMO – Resident Medical Officer

RN – Registered Nurse

RTA – Road Traffic Accident

SCI – Spinal Cord Injury

SDH – Subdural Hematoma

SOP – Standard Operating Procedures

SSC – Surgical Safety Checklist

STAT – “stat” is an abbreviation of the Latin Word Statim Means Immediately

SVD – Single Vessel Disease

TDS – ‘ter die sumendum’ means 3 times a day

TL – Team Leader

UF – Ultra Filtration

UHID – Unique Hospital Identification Number

USG – Ultrasonography

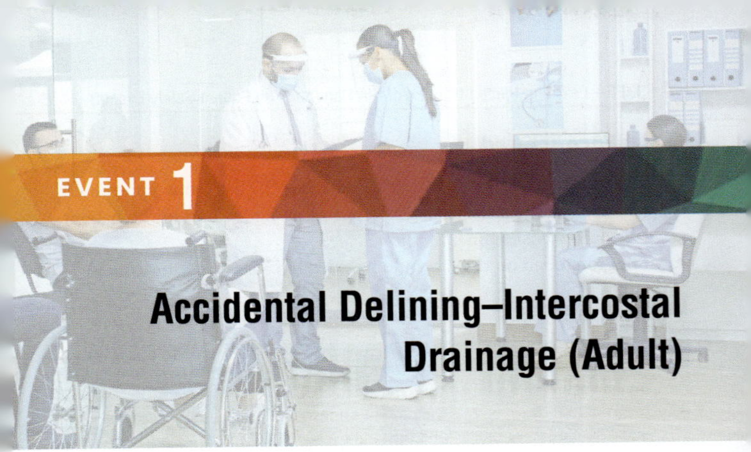

EVENT 1

Accidental Delining–Intercostal Drainage (Adult)

EVENT NO.	PSE/001/092022
IPSG RELATED TO	None

CASE STUDY DESCRIPTION

A 44-year-old male patient had been admitted after a road traffic accident with fractured ribs and pneumothorax. An intercostal drainage (ICD) tube was placed in the fourth intercostal space, in the mid-axillary region. The patient's fractured rib was stable with no flail chest. The ICD was connected to an underwater seal drainage bag. As per the protocol, the night nurse changed the ICD bag on day two at around 7:45 am. The thoracic surgeon came to see the patient early as he had to go to the operation theater (OT). When he visited the patient, the night nurse was handing over to the morning nurse. As soon as he saw the patient, the surgeon raised alarm and said, "Thank God, I came at the right time. Else, my patient would have arrested due to tension pneumothorax." The air vent of the ICD bag was not open.

Positive Outcomes

- The surgeon on his visit identified the air vent of the ICD bag was closed after changing the bag.
- The time between the error and the surgeon's visit was short so the patient did not develop serious complications.

Errors Encountered

- The nurses did not open the air vent of the ICD bag, which prevented the air from the pneumothorax from escaping leading to the patient developing tension pneumothorax.
- If not identified on time it could have led to catastrophic outcomes.

Lessons Learned

For nurse	For nurse educator	For nurse administrator
• The nurses must double-check the entire drainage system from the patient to the bag to ensure they have not missed anything after changing the bag. • During handover, both nurses must check the patient together. Entire length of all the tubes should be checked thoroughly.	• Train nurses to check the patient's lines and tubes in their entirety by both the nurses during handover. • Bedside training and on-the-spot corrections of errors must be done. • Ensure bedside handover of all the patients. • Convert such incidents into scenario-based learning.	• Implement the use of a handover checklist during nursing handover in every shift. • Critical procedure specific check points should be highlighted in the handover checklist • Double checking by two nurses during ICD bag change to be implemented. • Conduct root cause analysis and implement preventive measures like checking for column movement in the ICD drainage.

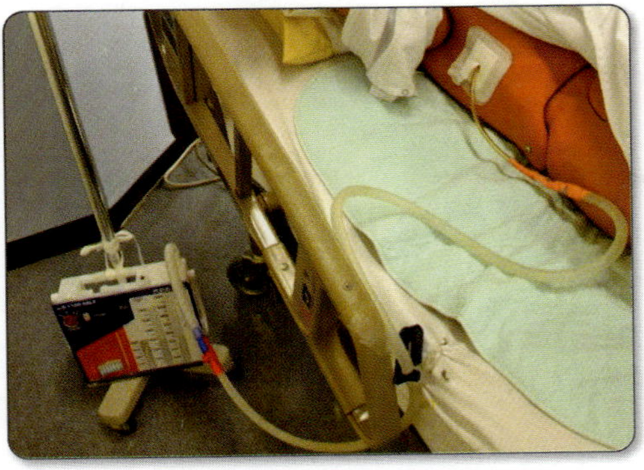

Figure 1 Patient with intercostal drainage bag

Event-Based Learning Summary

In the care of patients with chest tube drainages, patient safety takes precedence. To safeguard their well-being, conduct frequent assessments of the chest tube system, educate patients and their families on the importance of noninterference, secure connections diligently, exercise caution during patient's mobilization, and ensure clear labeling and comprehensive documentation. Effective communication with the healthcare team, adherence to established protocols, and swift action in response to accidental dislodgements are vital.

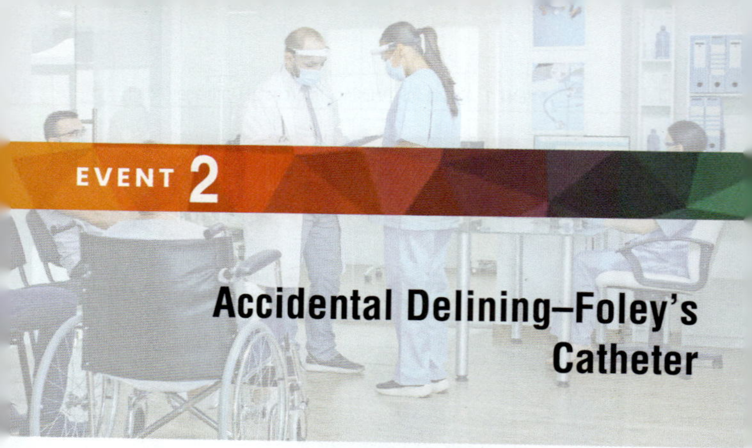

EVENT 2

Accidental Delining–Foley's Catheter

EVENT NO.	PSE/002/092022
IPSG RELATED TO	None

CASE STUDY DESCRIPTION

Mr Suresh was admitted to the medical ward on July 6, 2022 with the diagnosis of acute cerebrovascular accident (CVA) with right-sided hemiplegia. The patient was on a finger restraint in his left hand. The patient became restless and pulled out the silicone Foley's catheter. Mild bleeding was present at urethra which stopped soon after. The assigned nurse escalated the matter to the nursing supervisor.

Positive Outcomes

- Immediately assessed the patient's condition.
- A urology opinion was obtained.
- Re-catheterization was done.

Errors Encountered

- Nurses did not apply the restraint appropriately.
- Nurses did not monitor the restraint and the patient.
- The patient had to undergo a repeat catheterization.

Lessons Learned

For nurse	For nurse educator	For nurse administrator
• Ensure application of correct restraints. • Ensure catheters are secured. • Patient on restraint must be closely monitored.	• Train nurses on handling of patients on restraints. • Discussion by nurse trainers on such incidents, their root cause and corrective actions. • CNE on care of patient on restraints.	• Review policy, effectiveness of restraints and patient status on restrained patients regularly. • Conduct root cause analysis and corrective and preventive actions (CAPA) of such incidents. • Ensure right staffing

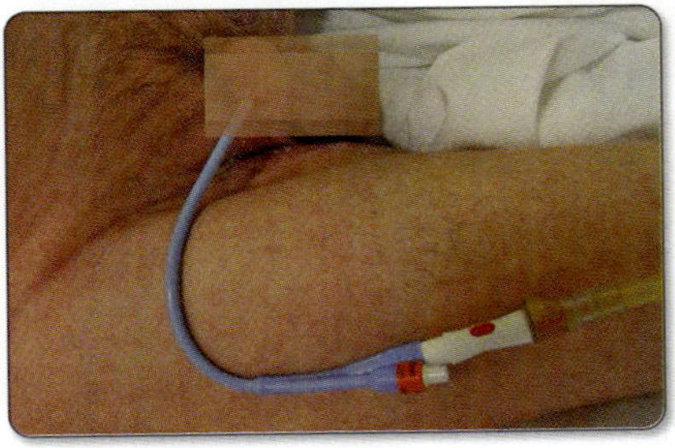

Figure 2 Male patient pulled out the silicone Foley's catheter

Event-Based Learning Summary

Ensuring the security of Foley's catheters is important for patient safety. Regularly assess the catheter, its placement, and the drainage system for any sign of dislodgement or incorrect positioning. Confirm that the catheter is correctly inserted, with the balloon properly inflated and secured. Educate both the patient and their caregivers about the catheter's significance and the importance of refraining from fidgeting it. Properly secure the catheter with nonstress loop, avoiding excessive tension. Employ clear labeling of connections, document diligently, and maintain open communication with the healthcare team to address any concern promptly. Consistently follow hospital protocols and guidelines for catheter management, and be prepared to take immediate action in case of accidental dislodgement. Preventing such incidents is fundamental to protect patient from injury and infection.

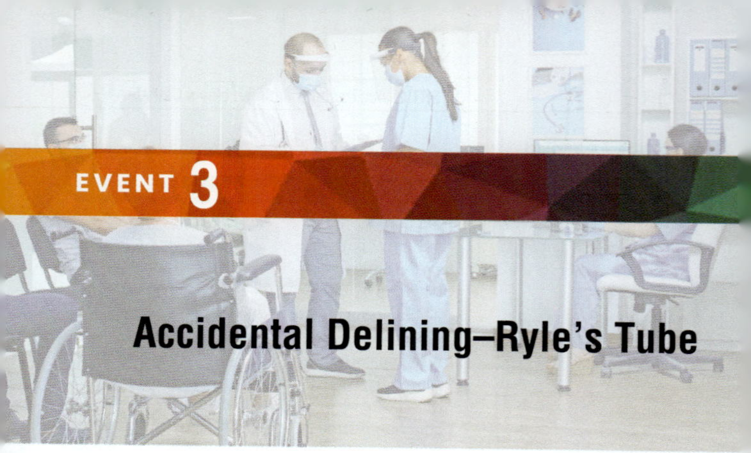

EVENT 3

Accidental Delining–Ryle's Tube

EVENT NO.	PSE/003/092022
IPSG RELATED TO	None

CASE STUDY DESCRIPTION

On May 18, 2022 in the male surgical ward, Mr Arun, a 65-year-old patient was admitted with complaints of vomiting and abdominal pain. He was diagnosed with acute pancreatitis. He had a previous history of cerebrovascular accident (CVA) and was on nil per orally (NPO) due to severe gastric pain and vomiting. He was receiving physiotherapy. On third day, i.e., May 20, 2022 morning at 8:15 am during physiotherapy, the Ryle's tube was accidentally expelled from its position which was inserted for aspiration of gastric content.

Positive Outcomes

- Immediately, the nurse reassessed the patient without any delay.
- The patient did not have any injury.
- Patient vitals were stable.
- The patient was kept in a comfortable position (Fowler's position).
- The assigned nurse immediately informed the incident to the treating consultant.
- New Ryle's tube was inserted without further delay to prevent further complication.

Errors Encountered

- The physiotherapist had not checked with the nurses regarding any safety precautions they needed to follow.
- The assigned nurse also did not inform the physiotherapist of the risk of delining.
- The assigned nurse did not offer help.
- The patient could have been explained before initiating the physiotherapy.

Lessons Learned

For nurse	For nurse educator	For nurse administrator
• Two care providers need to be with patients during physiotherapy when such risks are likely to occur. • Double-check the proper method of securing the Ryle's tube. • Ensure that the tube is securely anchored to the patient's nose to prevent excess tube movement and stressed loop is maintained. • Periodic assessment of the nasogastric (NG) tube placement.	• Nurses to be taught well on the importance of patient education in their care. • Involvement of patient and his/her companions in education and care. • Focus on bedside trainings. • Train nurses on expected accidents with NG tube (Ryles Tube).	• Conduct root cause analysis and implement corrective and preventive actions (CAPA) for such incidents. • Collaborate with physiotherapy department to ensure that the physiotherapist check with the assigned nurse for any safety concerns.

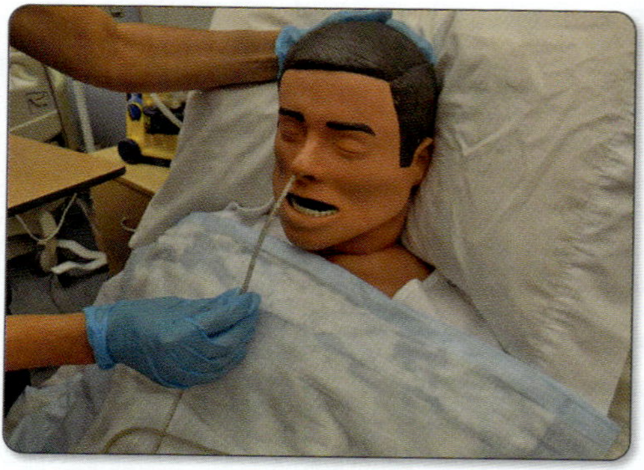

Figure 3 Accidentally expelled nasogastric tube

Event-Based Learning Summary

When tending to patients with Ryle's tube, the possibility of accidental dislodgement should always be considered. Essential steps to preserve the tube's integrity include the proper tube securement, nonstress loop to avoid tension, frequent placement assessment and report concerns immediately. Patients and caregivers should be educated about the importance of not tampering with the tube and reporting concerns promptly. Ensure that the incoming and outgoing nurses check all tubes including Ryle's tube during shift handover. Immediate action should be taken in case of accidental dislodgement. Preventing such incidents is fundamental for prevention of complication like aspiration.

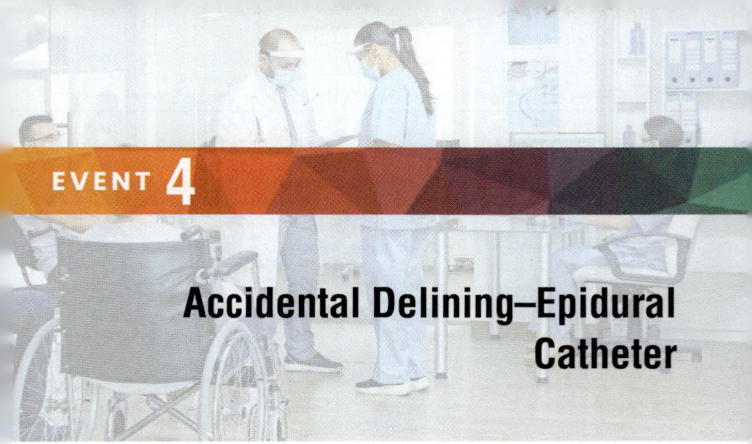

EVENT 4

Accidental Delining–Epidural Catheter

EVENT NO.	PSE/004/092022
IPSG RELATED TO	None

CASE STUDY DESCRIPTION

A 34-year-old male was admitted to the hospital with the diagnosis of right lower limb multiligament injury. The patient had undergone surgery on December 29, 2021. The patient had an accidental removal of the epidural catheter on the same day.

Positive Outcomes

- The patient was not harmed.
- There was no immediate neurological consequences.
- No fragments of the catheter were retained.

Error Encountered

- The patient had accidental removal of the epidural catheter while positioning.
- The team had not taken extra care during positioning.

Lessons Learned

For nurse	For nurse educator	For nurse administrator
• Checking the placement of the epidural line during handover from OT staff. • Provide instructions to the patient before moving. • Assigned nurse to ensure that he/she has received training on care of epidural line.	Training of nurses on "Care of Patient with Epidural Line" should include: • Features of epidural line • Indications and Contraindications • Positioning of patient with epidural lines • Potential complications and its preventions. • Essential assessments of patient and epidural line • Care and dressing of epidural lines • Handling of epidural infusions • Assessment of training needs based on incidents reported and facilitate training.	• Ensure clear guidelines on managing the epidural catheter is documented in nursing SOPs. • Designate a safety officer to take rounds and check high risk patient, wherever possible. • Plan regular nursing audits/checks to ensure that patient safety guidelines are effectively implemented.

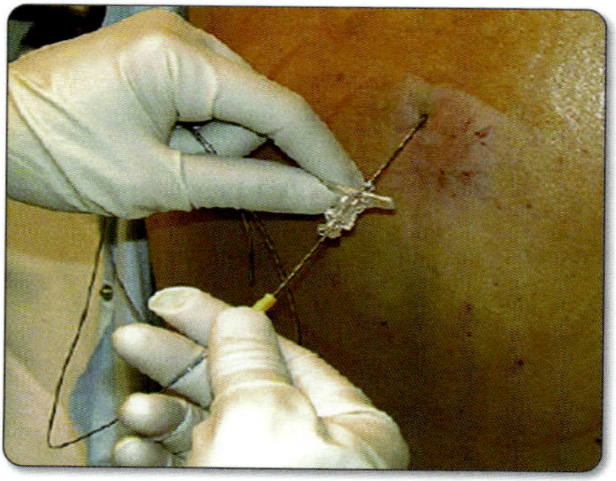

Figure 4 Epidural Catheter

Event-Based Learning Summary

Ensuring the safety and efficacy of pain management for patients with epidural catheters is a top priority. To prevent accidental dislodgement, follow these steps:

Regularly assess the catheter's placement and securement, being vigilant for signs of dislodgement or misalignment. Educate both the patient and their caregivers about the catheter's importance, stressing the need to avoid any manipulation and promptly report changes in sensation and position.

Secure the catheter with suitable techniques and devices to prevent accidental dislodgement, making sure it is firmly anchored without excess tension. Clearly label all catheter connections to avoid accidental disconnections, particularly during care transitions. During patient mobilization, take special care to secure and support the catheter to prevent tension on the tubing.

Accurate documentation and open communication within the healthcare team are essential. Familiarize yourself with hospital protocols for epidural catheter management and adhere to best practices. In the event of accidental dislodgement, follow established protocols for prompt assistance to ensure timely intervention, i.e., escalating same to the doctor without delay.

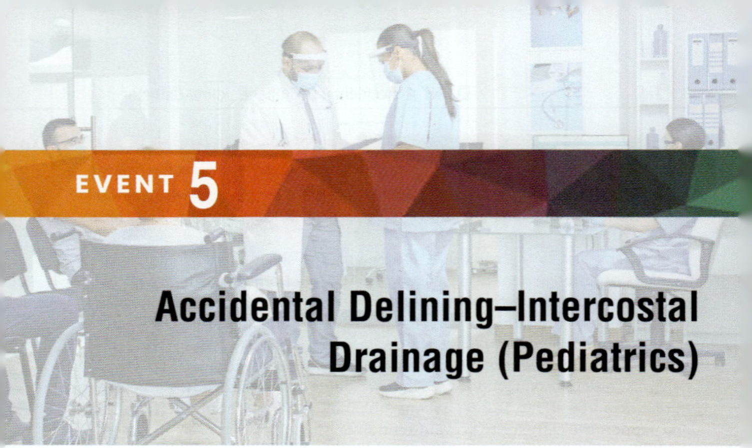

EVENT 5

Accidental Delining–Intercostal Drainage (Pediatrics)

EVENT NO.	PSE/005/092022
IPSG RELATED TO	None

CASE STUDY DESCRIPTION

A 3-year-old child was admitted to the pediatric intensive care unit on 19/04/2022 with a history of fall from height. The child was on a ventilator and had intercostal drainage (ICD) tubes bilaterally. On 3rd day of hospitalization, the child was extubated and put on noninvasive ventilation without sedation. There was an accidental removal of ICD tube while securing the ICD drain.

Positive Outcomes

- Immediate identification of the delining.
- Sealed the ICD opening by pressure dressing.
- Suturing of the ICD opening was done, and an X-ray was taken to check for pneumothorax.
- The child's vital parameters were normal.

Errors Encountered

- ICD tubes was removed accidentally because the child was not sedated adequately (sedatives could not be provided due to postextubation).
- The child was not restrained and monitored by the nurse.

Lessons Learned

For nurse	For nurse educator	For nurse administrator
• To have adequate procedure preparedness, especially with Pediatrics. High risk category must be handled carefully. • Restrain the child if required, after taking consent from the parents. Or better, allow one parent to be present during such procedures to hold and restrain the child.	• Train nurses on parents' education. • Induct PICU nurses on troubleshooting and handling complications related to intercostal drains. • Assess training needs based on incidents reported and facilitate training.	• Develop policy on pediatric patient restraints. • Privileged nurses to be deployed to handle high-risk category cases in pediatric ICU. • Conduct root cause analysis as well as corrective and preventive actions (CAPA) of such incidents.

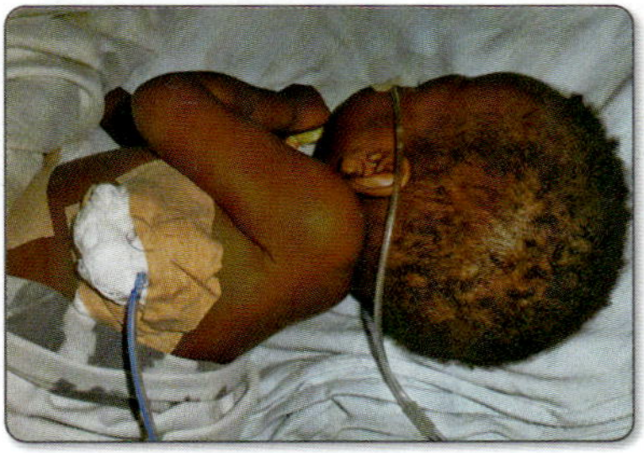

Figure 5 Child with intercostal drainage

Event-Based Learning Summary

When caring for pediatric patients with intercostal drainage tubes, ensuring their safety is paramount. Key measures to reduce the risk of accidental dislodgement include constant supervision, proper securement with pediatric-specific devices, and applying secure but not overly tight dressings. Educate parents or caregivers about the importance of not disturbing the tube and recognizing signs of dislodgement or complications. Maintain a child-centered approach, explaining the tube's presence in an age-appropriate manner and minimizing mobility risks. Document diligently and respond promptly to dislodgement by following hospital protocols and notifying the medical team. In complex cases, seek the expertise of pediatric specialists to address unique needs. Above all, prioritize the child's safety and provide meticulous care to prevent complications. Your commitment is pivotal to their safety and recovery.

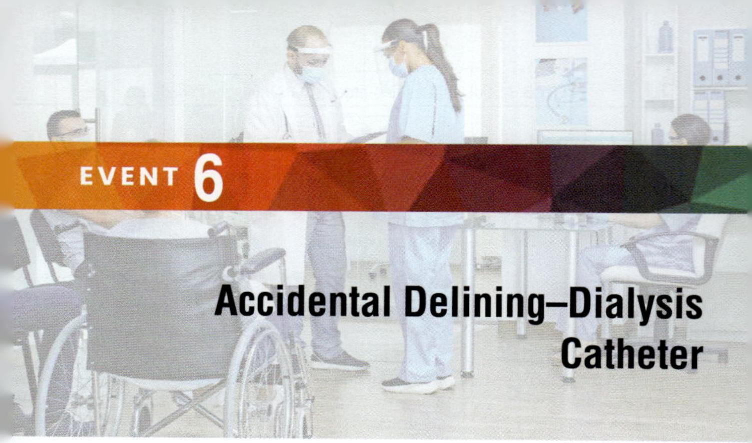

EVENT 6

Accidental Delining–Dialysis Catheter

EVENT NO.	PSE/006/092022
IPSG RELATED TO	None

CASE STUDY DESCRIPTION

A 55-year-old female got admitted with chronic kidney disease (CKD), hypertension (HTN), and diabetes mellitus (DM). The patient was on hemodialysis through Diacath inserted via the femoral route and was in situ. The patient had a CT scan planned, for which she was shifted to the CT scan department. At the CT scan department, RN was busy taking another patient's vitals; the handover was very brief, wasn't complete, and was not documented. While taking the patient from bed to trolley, her Dialysis catheter or Diacath was accidentally pulled, causing her severe pain and agony. When the staff removed the bed sheet, she realized the patient had an invasive femoral line. She was assessed for bleeding and swelling, which was not present. When the patient returned to the room, the incident escalated that no handover regarding the patient's invasive line was received in the CT scan department and could have caused accidental de-lining of the same. The consultant was informed about the incident and re-evaluated the Diacath for its correct position.

Positive Outcomes

- Immediate escalation of the incidence was done.
- The gap was addressed in the missed opportunity of handover, which gave a platform to improve the process.

Errors Encountered

- Registered nurse (RN) missed giving details about the patient, especially about the invasive lines of the patient.
- Nurses missed the handover opportunities during interdepartmental transfers.

Lessons Learned

For nurse	For nurse educator	For nurse administrator
• If occupied, RN should wait for proper handover, and RN taking the handover should also be equally vigilant to take effective takeover. • The transition of care is a critical junction, where inadequate handover can lead to patient harm. • Ensure complete and documented handover. • Explain the procedure to the patient before starting.	• Train nurses on the complete handover process and inculcate the practice of documented handover. • Train nurses to emphasize on the safety aspects of the patient during handover including the presence of all the lines and tubes	• To include intra-department transfers nursing documentation notes as a mandate in nursing documentation SOPs. • Prepare a transfer checklist for diagnostic procedures of all admitted patients including all safety aspects.

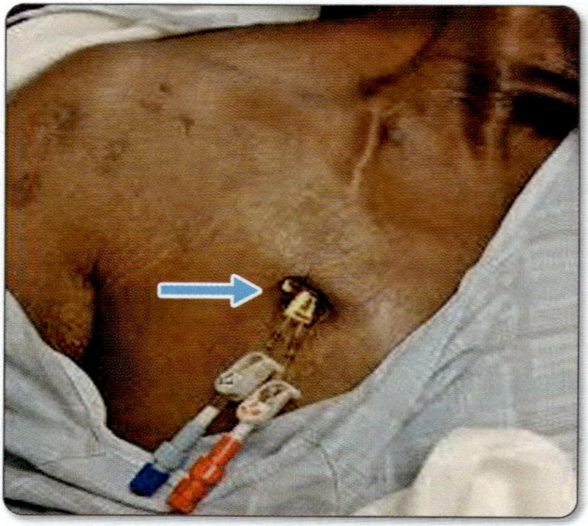

Figure 6 Removal of dialysis catheter

Event-Based Learning Summary

Caring for patients with dialysis catheter demands unwavering attention to prevent accidental dislodgement, ensuring their safety and the effectiveness of hemodialysis. Essential measures to reduce the risk of dislodgement include frequent assessment, confirming proper insertion, educating patients on non-interference, using securement devices, and clearly labeling connections. During patient mobility, ensure the catheter's adequate support without tension. Thorough documentation and seamless communication within the healthcare team are vital. Adherence to protocols and immediate response to dislodgement are critical for the patient's well-being. Preventing accidental dislodgement is fundamental for delivering quality renal replacement therapy.

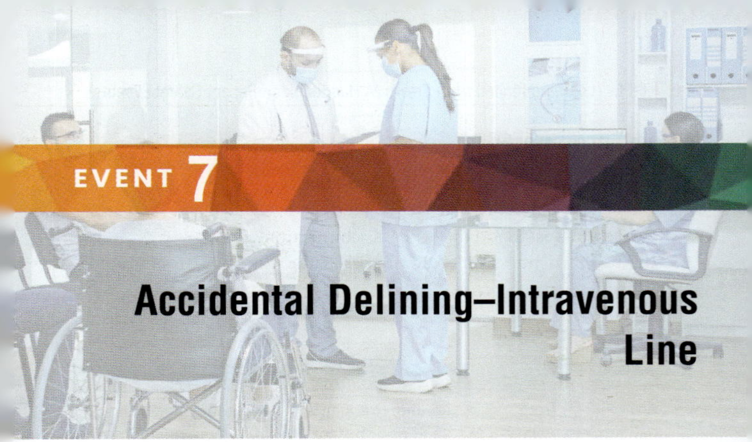

EVENT 7

Accidental Delining–Intravenous Line

EVENT NO.	PSE/007/092022
IPSG RELATED TO	None

CASE STUDY DESCRIPTION

The nurses frequently made rounds on patients in a particular hospital to assess their needs. But there was also an increased number of complaints from the patient side that the nurses were disturbing patients to check vitals, lines etc., during the night. Hence, the management decided to stop the nurses from making frequent rounds at night.

During the night shift, the staff nurse connected 0.45% DNS for Mr Salman, who was 73-year-old admitted with acute gastroenteritis. The nurse said she would come in-between to check on him, but the patient told the nurse not to disturb him as he wanted to sleep. After 4 hours, the nurse checked the infusion and was going to connect the next intravenous (IV) fluid. As she inspected the three-way connection of the IV tip, she found that it was disconnected, and the fluid was spilled on the floor. The bedsheet was filled with blood. She immediately informed the on-duty doctor, checked the vital signs, and sent blood samples to rule out blood and electrolyte loss.

Positive Outcome

None.

Errors Encountered

- Accidental disconnection of the IV line.
- The patient did not receive the IV fluid.
- The patient lost blood due to IV disconnection.
- The assigned nurse failed to check on the patient with continuous infusion.

Lessons Learned

For nurse	For nurse educator	For nurse administrator
• Any requests from patients/attendants must be considered only if it is safe for the patient. • The nurse should explain to the patient and attendant that she has to come in quietly to check that the IV site is ok and the fluid is infusing correctly. • Use correct securement method. • Use extension tubing to minimize catheter movement and gain more adhesive surface area. • Ensure that the three way stopcocks are secured tightly; use IV sets with luer lock connection.	• Routine checking of vitals or disturbing a well-resting patient is not required, however educate nurses that the clinical rounds need to be individualized and need-based. • Reasons for accidental delining and disconnection including preventive actions must be part of the nurses training.	• Ensure mandatory patient safety rounds for patient's needing frequent assessment. • Implement frequent rounds using the 4 Ps (Pain, Potty, Position, and Possession) to reduce patient harm. • Conduct root cause analysis as well as corrective and preventive actions (CAPA) for such incidents.

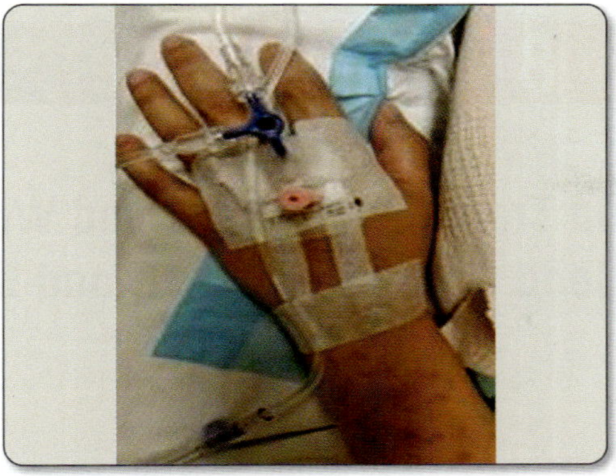

Figure 7 Intravenous line

Event-Based Learning Summary

When tending to patients with peripheral IV lines, unwavering vigilance is essential to prevent accidental dislodgement and ensure uninterrupted access for medications and fluids. It is worth noting that more than 80% of the patients might rely on peripheral IV access. Key steps to minimize the risk include regular assessment, proper insertion and site selection, patient education, securement techniques, clear labeling of connections, and thoughtful consideration during patient mobility. Accurate documentation and open communication with the healthcare team are crucial, as is adherence to hospital protocols and immediate action in the event of dislodgement. Preventing accidental dislodgement is pivotal for maintaining treatment effectiveness and patient comfort.

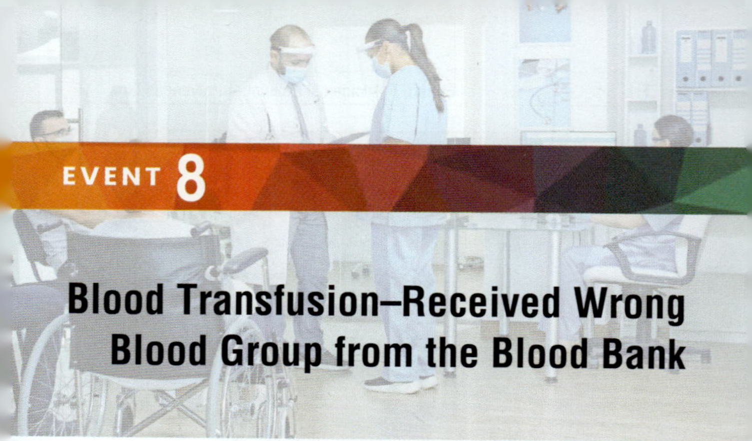

EVENT 8

Blood Transfusion–Received Wrong Blood Group from the Blood Bank

EVENT NO.	PSE/008/092022
IPSG RELATED TO	None

CASE STUDY DESCRIPTION

A 60-year-old male was diagnosed to have cancer prostate. The doctor advised transfusing one unit of the O +ve blood. Staff sent crossmatching and requisition forms to the blood bank. The housekeeping staff went to the blood bank, received the blood, and handed it over to the assigned nurse. An assigned nurse while cross checking found that the blood received was A +ve and informed to the shift Team Leader (TL). However the TL neither instructed the junior nurse to send it back to the blood bank nor advised to raise the event. The nurse took the photographs of the blood bag and sent them to the resident doctor, who was at home, for verification of the blood bag details. He checked the details and instructed her to transfuse blood. Staff transfused blood. The supervisor on rounds discovered the patient was receiving A +ve blood instead of O +ve blood and the blood transfusion was stopped immediately.

Positive Outcome

None.

Errors Encountered

- There was a total breakdown of all protocols related to safe blood transfusion.
- Though the error was found, the senior staff in the department failed to escalate it to anyone.
- The junior nurse simply followed the senior one without applying her mind.
- Communication with the doctor was through WhatsApp and shared photographs of labels, which are not acceptable protocols.
- The doctor also failed to verify the critical details of the patient, and the blood bag.

Lessons Learned

For nurse	For nurse educator	For nurse administrator
• Have the confidence to escalate the mistake than trusting seniors. We cannot undo the harm that would reach the patient. • Before transfusing the blood, the staff should cross-check the product details clearly with that of cross-matching slip and the file. • No verbal orders are to be carried out.	• Good to develop a protocol to follow 'CUS' for patient safety— C = I am concerned U = I am uncomfortable S = It is a safety issue. • Train and highlight double-checking done by another nurse which need to be documented and signed. • Sensitize nurses that they are individually accountable for patient harm if there is non-compliance.	• To insist on adhering to policies where the doctor should be physically present and document the compatibility of the blood products and must write in the progress notes. • Without this step being done diligently, nurse should not be allowed to administer the blood products. • Blood transfusion is a highly regulated service in the hospital. Ensure the first check is done by the blood bank.

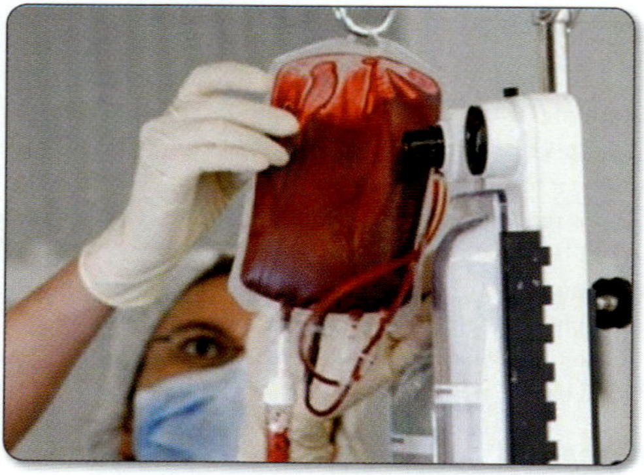

Figure 8 Blood transfusion

Event-Based Learning Summary

As nurses, you hold a pivotal role in preventing blood transfusion errors from reaching the patient. Rigorous patient verification, utilizing barcode technology, and team-based cross-checks are vital steps in ensuring patient safety. Confirming blood group compatibility, scrutinizing labels, and voicing concerns when necessary is essential for preventing mistakes. Obtaining informed consent, conducting bedside verifications, and maintaining vigilant monitoring are key aspects of this process. Reporting near misses and fostering a culture of safety within your healthcare setting further enhance patient safety. In this shared responsibility, nurse's diligence and commitment are instrumental in delivering safe and reliable patient care.

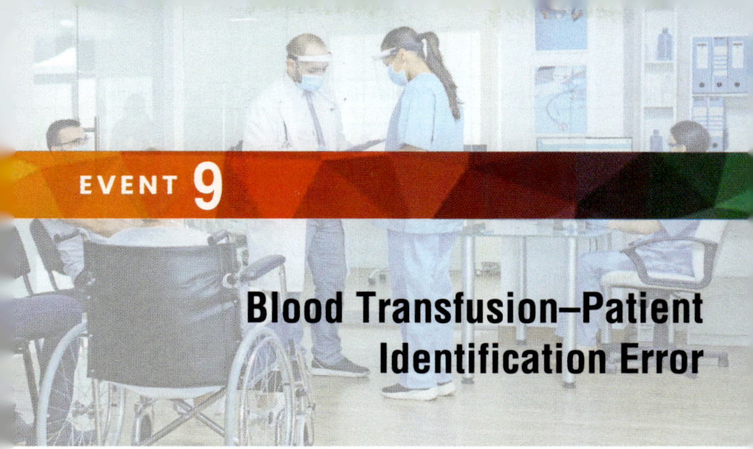

EVENT 9

Blood Transfusion–Patient Identification Error

EVENT NO.	PSE/009/092022
IPSG RELATED TO	IPSG 1 – Correct Patient Identification

CASE STUDY DESCRIPTION

Mr Mahesh, a patient was admitted to twin sharing room. Doctor advised for blood transfusion to the patient. Mr Sumit, the patient in the next bed, was also advised for a blood transfusion.

The nurses received a call from the blood bank that the blood bag for Mr Mahesh will be available after 2 hours. Also they asked to send GDA within 15 minutes to collect the blood for Mr Sumit.

As per the conversation, blood bank is supposed to send Mr Sumit's blood bag for transfusion, but the blood bank sent the bag for Mr Mahesh.

Team leader received the blood, assumed the same as per the conversation, and asked Mr Sumit's assigned staff to get verified by the doctor and start the transfusion for Mr Sumit, not realizing that this blood bag was sent for Mr Mahesh.

The doctor verified the blood bag and documented in Mr Sumit's notes. The assigned staff checked the vitals of Mr Sumit and started the blood transfusion.

After 30 minutes, when she came to check the vital signs, the patient complained of redness on the hands and itching all over the body.

Then she stopped the blood and informed the doctor. The doctor advised Inj. Dexamethazone and Inj. Avil, which the nurse administered.

Then nurse informed the blood bank of the same, and blood and urine samples were sent along with transfusion reaction form.

The blood bank also received it, but lost the sample, the blood bank asked the TL to send the repeat sample of Mr Mahesh. But TL was confused because blood was administered to Mr Sumit, and only then the mistake was identified.

Positive Outcome

None.

Error Encountered

There was total breakdown of safety protocols. The telephonic information should not have been relied upon. The safety protocols of initiating the blood transfusion was not adhered to.

Lessons Learned

For nurse	For nurse educator	For nurse administrator
• Use two identifiers during any procedure involving the patient. • This identification must be performed by the nurse administering the blood in the presence of another nurse by cross checking doctor's orders with the cross match slip and blood bag label. • When receiving telephonic information, perform Read-Back. • Include patient's name when explaining the procedure. • This identification must be performed by the person administering the blood in the presence of another staff.	• Train nurses to have final double-checking at the bedside just before starting the transfusion. • Regular training on the blood transfusion policy (include handling potential complications) and patient safety goals. • Disseminate the learnings from these incidents to other staffs.	• Institute policy on verbal order to include situation and procedures where verbal orders are accepted. • Blood bank must carry a proper check before sending the blood to the IP areas. • Incorporate Barcode system to confirm identity between wristband and blood bag label.

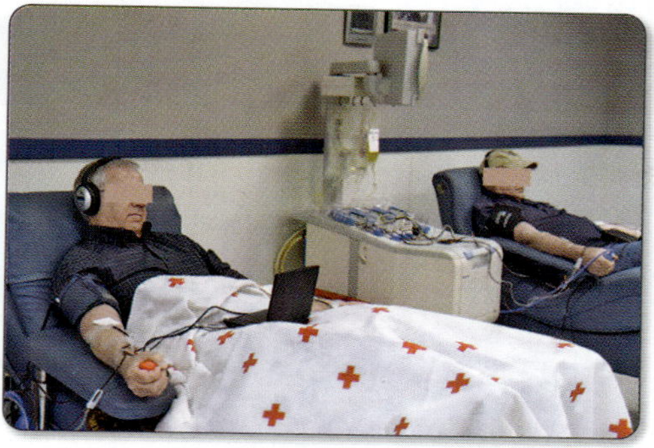

Figure 9 Blood transfusion in twin sharing room for two patients

Event-Based Learning Summary

Nurses play a vital role in averting patient identification errors during blood transfusion. To ensure patient safety, it is crucial to implement a two-step verification process, use barcode technology, engage another healthcare professional for verification, involve the patient, and meticulously compare the blood bag label with the patient's identity. Verify orders, document carefully, maintain open team communication, obtain patient's consent, and stay updated through regular training. Promote a culture of safety where concerns are voiced and errors are considered to create opportunities for improvement as it is the key to patient safety. These measures collectively mitigate the risk of identification-related errors and bolster patient safety during transfusions.

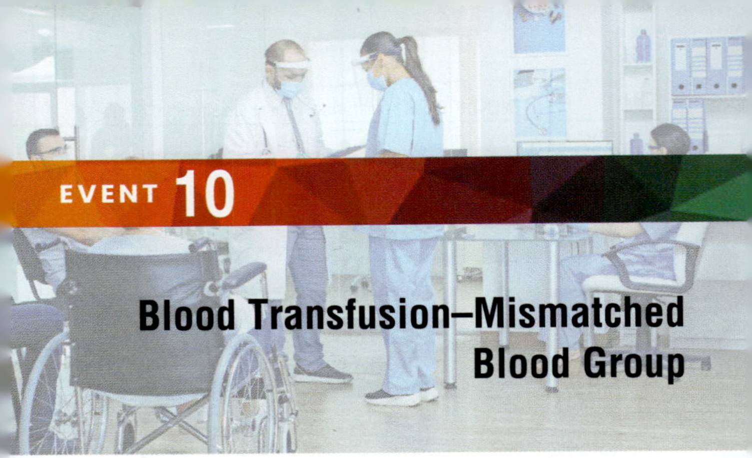

EVENT 10

Blood Transfusion–Mismatched Blood Group

EVENT NO.	PSE/010/092022
IPSG RELATED TO	IPSG 1 – Correct Patient Identification

CASE STUDY DESCRIPTION

A 26-year-old lady was diagnosed with fibroid uterus and underwent laparoscopic surgery. There was postoperative blood loss following the surgery. On her second postoperative day, the treating doctor requested a blood transfusion for the patient. The nurse attending the patient asks the attendants to bring two units of O +ve blood from the blood bank. After the attendants returned with the blood, the attending nurse forgot to take the blood approval from the treating consultant and immediately transfused the blood to the patient without cross-checking it, as the patient's blood pressure was falling. As the nurse started transfusing the blood, she noticed that the patient started developing rashes all over her body, and was complaining of breathing difficulty. The nurse stopped the transfusion, and called the doctor immediately. The doctor advised her to administer Inj. Avil 2 mL, which was administered. The patient went into anaphylactic shock and was immediately transferred to the Critical Care Unit (CCU). It was found that the patient was transfused with a B +ve group of blood instead of O +ve.

Positive Outcome

None.

Errors Encountered

- The patient family should not be asked to bring the blood.
- The nurse had not correctly cross-checked with the patient record, crossmatch slip, and the patient.
- Before dispatching the blood, the blood bank should have cross-checked twice along with the patient's blood group.
- The nurse did not follow the double-check procedure with the doctor at the bedside.

Lessons Learned

For nurse	For nurse educator	For nurse administrator
• A complete written order for blood transfusion must be available before the nurse starts the transfusion. • Every nurse must focus on following all the steps of the blood transfusion procedure.	• Train nurses on transfusion protocols. • Discussing the incident, root cause, corrective and preventive actions with staff.	• Documented SOPs which clearly mention that before dispatching the blood, the blood bank of the hospital should cross-check twice along with the patient's blood group. • Institute the policy where a senior nurse like incharge/nurse supervisor does a second verification at the bedside. • Include verbal confirmation with the patient/relative regarding the patient blood type as an additional safety mechanism to avoid transfusion error.

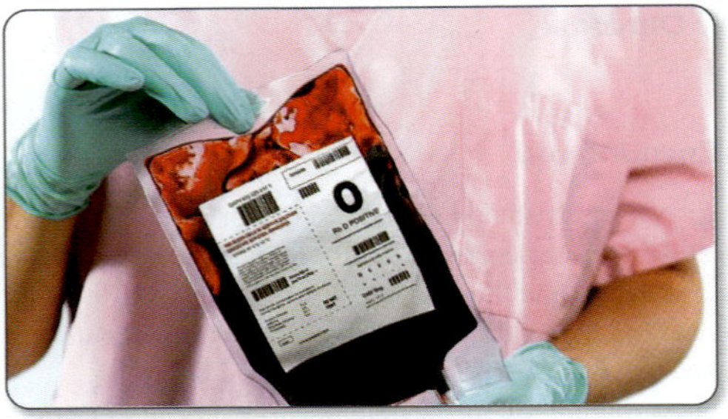

Figure 10 Blood transfusion with O +ve

Event-Based Learning Summary

Preventing blood transfusion errors, especially those arising from using the wrong blood bag, is paramount for patient safety. Robust measures are essential. Verify the blood bag label meticulously, employ a two-step verification process, and utilize barcode scanning technology when available. Engage another healthcare professional for independent verification, actively involve the patient, and check blood compatibility. Ensure accurate labeling, the correctness of blood orders, and maintain careful documentation. Foster a culture of open communication and always secure informed patient consent. Ongoing training and education are crucial for staying updated with best practices. These measures collectively reduce the risk of using the wrong blood bag, upholding patient safety during transfusions.

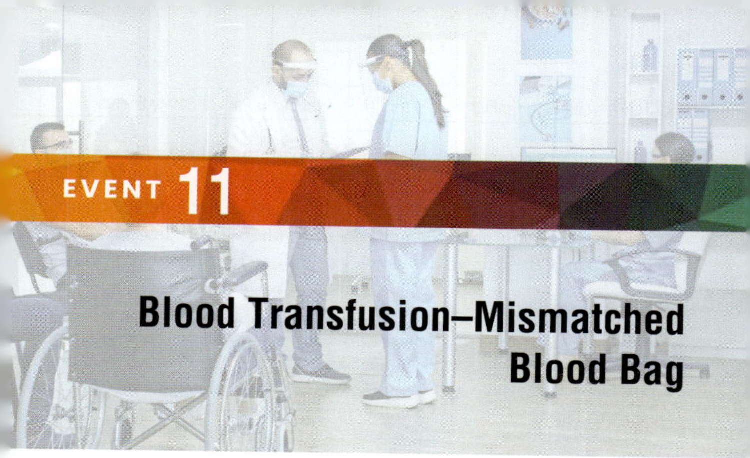

EVENT 11

Blood Transfusion–Mismatched Blood Bag

EVENT NO.	PSE/011/092022
IPSG RELATED TO	None

CASE STUDY DESCRIPTION

Mrs Nita was admitted to the General Ward at 3:50 pm, the nurse sent O +ve blood requisition to the blood bank. But the blood bank technician sent B +ve blood. The RMO checked the blood bag and wrote details in the doctor's progress notes. The staff nurse checked the blood and the notes and started the blood transfusion. Subsequently the staff nurse checked the IPD file, and found that the patient was O +ve and the blood bag was of B +ve. Immediately, the nurse stopped the blood transfusion and informed the respective consultant, who advised Inj. Hydrocort 100 mg, IV stat. Later on, the blood bag was returned to the blood bank.

Positive Outcomes

- Immediate action was taken by the nurse by stopping the blood transfusion and informing the consultant.
- Administration of Inj. Hydrocortizone as per consultant's order.

Errors Encountered

- Blood bank technician did not correlate the blood bag details with blood requisition.
- Nurse did not cross-check the blood bag with the patient's IPD file.

- RMO did not cross-check the blood bag with the patient's file for the blood group report.
- Nurse failed to reconfirm the patient's blood group just before starting the blood transfusion in the presence of another senior nurse.

There was a total breakdown in following safe blood transfusion protocols.

Lessons Learned

For nurse	For nurse educator	For nurse administrator
• The blood bag details (Patient name, UHID, blood group, Expiry date) must be checked. • These identifiers must be matched with the same information in the patient's file and cross-matched report and patient identification band. • Involve patient in identification process wherever it is possible. • Ensure that two healthcare professional must do the verification at patient bedside.	• Train nurses on Blood Transfusion SOP. • Reiterate on Patient identification. • Include blood transfusion policy in nurse's induction training. • Assess training needs based on audits and incidents reported and facilitate training as required.	• Create a robust policy for blood transfusion involving blood bank, Nursing and medical departments • Conduct root cause analysis and corrective and preventive actions (CAPA) for such incidents. • Plan to conduct random audits to check for adherence to safety protocols related to blood transfusion.

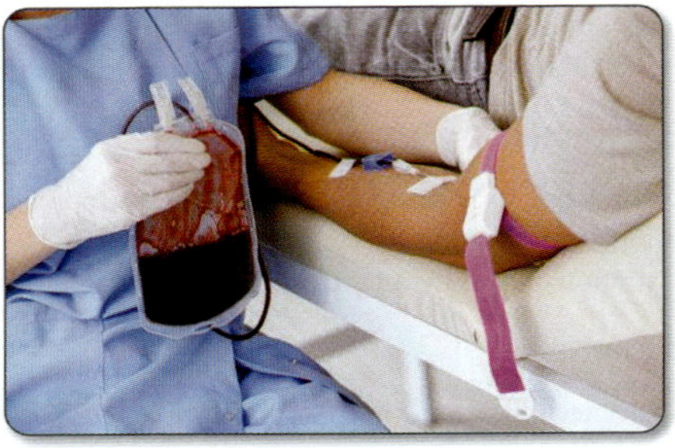

Figure 11 Blood transfusion stopped immediately

Event-Based Learning Summary

In the realm of patient care, it is imperative that nurses prioritize patient safety, especially during blood transfusions. Always double-check patient details such as names, and UHID to ensure they match the ID band, blood form, label on the blood bag. Verify the patient's blood group, reconfirm it before the transfusion begins, and include patient identifiers in every step of the process. If any discrepancies arise, take immediate action by stopping the transfusion, notifying the healthcare team, and following their guidance. Effective communication within the healthcare team is vital for error prevention and swift resolution. These precautions and commitment to patient safety are essential to prevent identification errors and ensure that the right blood products are administered to the right patients, ultimately saving lives and upholding the highest standard of care.

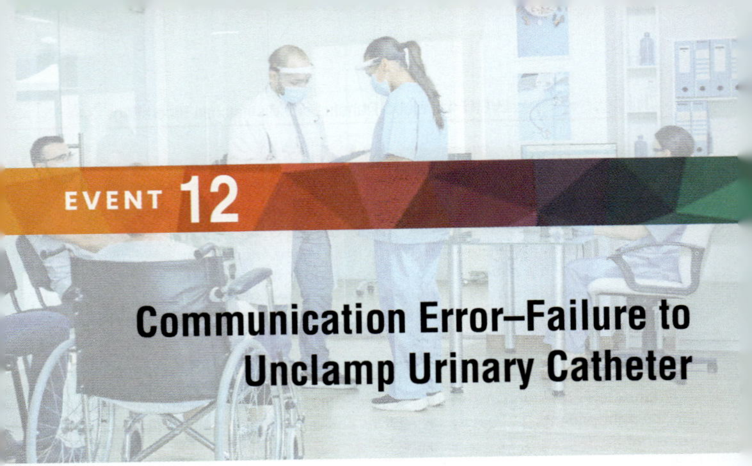

EVENT 12

Communication Error–Failure to Unclamp Urinary Catheter

EVENT NO.	PSE/012/092022
IPSG RELATED TO	IPSG 2 – Improve Effective Communication

CASE STUDY DESCRIPTION

The nurse was instructed to remove the urinary catheter after checking the sphincter control of the patient. A junior nurse clamped the catheter and did not give any instruction to the patient. The clamping of the catheter was not documented and not communicated during the handing-over session. When the next duty nurse took over, the patient called the nurse and said his bladder was full. Without assessing the patient, the nurse just called and reported to the doctor. The duty doctor came and identified the clamp and removed it.

Positive Outcome

None.

Errors Encountered

- The assigned nurse did not educate the patient on what was done and its purpose.
- Failure in documentation.
- Failure to communicate to the following shift staff.
- Failure to check the lines and tubes during handover.
- Failure to assess the patient before informing the doctor.

Lessons Learned

For nurse	For nurse educator	For nurse administrator
• Use structured communication tool for handover. • Document the handover. • Examine the patient and assess before reporting. • Incoming and outgoing nurses must check all the lines and tubes together during the handover.	• Train nurses on shift endorsement. • Focus on bedside training during in-service education. • Use such scenarios to conduct simulation-based learning (SBL).	• Audit shift endorsement process using a checklist. • Ensure such events are converted into learning session for all the nurses.

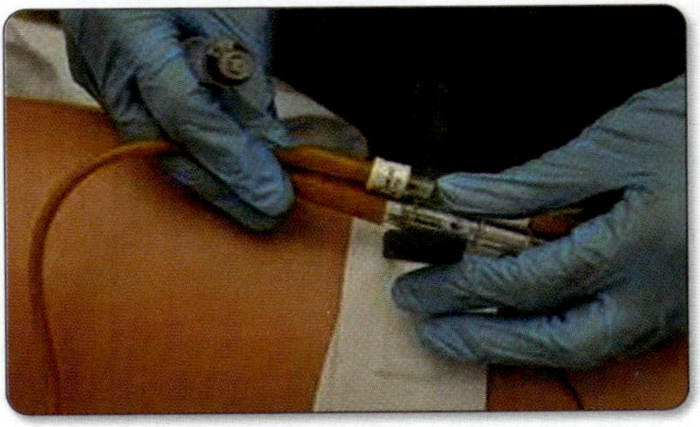

Figure 12 Failure to unclamp urinary catheter

Event-Based Learning Summary

Effective communication is the cornerstone of patient safety. To prevent errors like the one described, remember to educate patients about procedures, document changes in care, and communicate these changes during shift handovers. Regularly check equipment and lines to catch any issues, and always assess the patient's condition before involving a doctor. By following these steps, we can ensure patient understanding, maintain clear records, and prevent communication gaps, ultimately providing safer, high-quality care and preserving trust within the healthcare team.

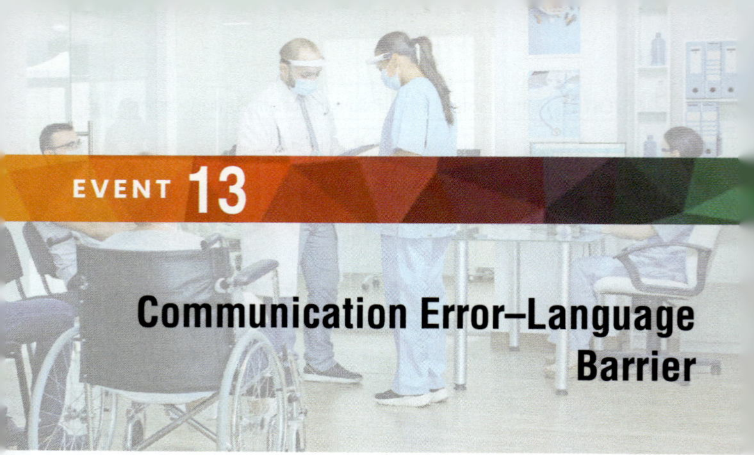

EVENT 13

Communication Error–Language Barrier

EVENT NO.	PSE/013/092022
IPSG RELATED TO	IPSG 2 – Improve Effective Communication

CASE STUDY DESCRIPTION

A 70-year-old woman came to the lab with the physician's order to do a routine urine examination. The student nurse gave a collection container to the patient and asked in Tamil to collect her urine sample. The patient went to rest room and collected her urine sample. When the lab technician performed the needed investigation, found that the sample was not urine; but water. The patient was given another container, and the urine specimen was obtained.

Positive Outcome

The student nurse gave the container and explained about the urine sample collection.

Error Encountered

The student nurse explained to the patient in Tamil. But it was misunderstood by the patient ***(Siru neer was mistaken as neer),*** and she collected water from the bucket.

Lessons Learned

For nurse	For nurse educator	For nurse administrator
• Communicate with the patient and family in the language that they understand. • Ask patient to Repeat Back the instructions. • Make use of communication chart/translator.	• Arrange language classes. • Train in-charge nurses on allocating the right staff to the patient with language barriers. • Train nurses to ask for help when they face patient with language barrier.	• To have signages being displayed to avoid language-related communication barrier. • Make available tools that can be used by nurses to make communication easier.

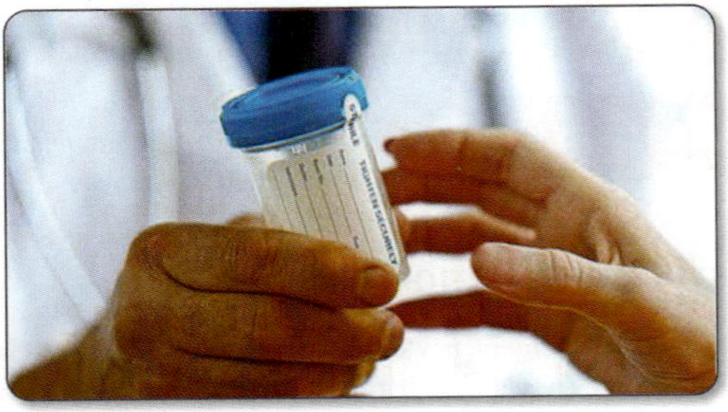

Figure 13 Nursing student giving urine sample bottle to female patient

Event-Based Learning Summary

In healthcare, effective communication is vital, especially when language barriers exist. To mitigate misunderstandings, communicate in the patient's language or use professional interpreters and visual aids. Encourage patients to confirm their understanding and offer language training for healthcare staff. Ensure that the right staff is assigned to patients with language barriers and utilize signage for clear communication. By following these steps, we can improve patient care, prevent errors, and create a more inclusive and safe healthcare environment for all.

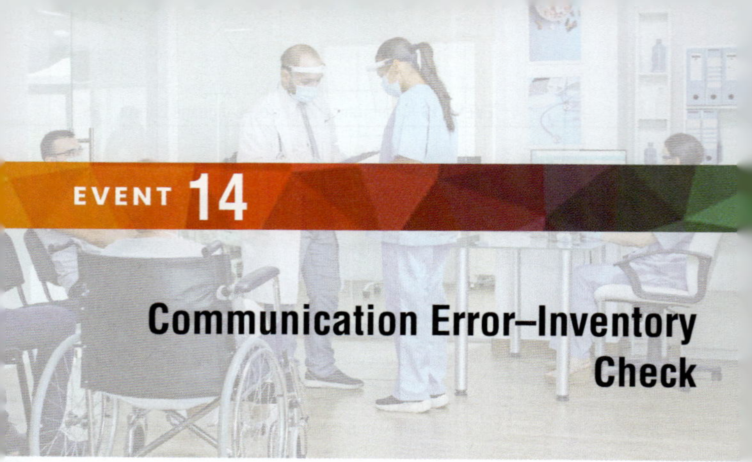

EVENT 14

Communication Error–Inventory Check

EVENT NO.	PSE/014/092022
IPSG RELATED TO	IPSG 2 – Improve Effective Communication

CASE STUDY DESCRIPTION

Mr Manish came to emergency department complaining of severe pain in the center of the chest and radiating to the left hand. While examining, the patient became unconscious and collapsed. The patient was shifted immediately to CCU. The doctors planned to intubate the patient and asked to be ready with the intubation tray. Positioned the patient and asked for a laryngoscope to insert an endotracheal tube. The nurse gave the laryngoscope, but it was not working. There was no battery inside the scope. It led to a delay in the procedure. Immediately the shift in-charge arranged laryngoscope from the emergency ward and intubated the patient. By that time the patient went into respiratory acidosis and had further complications.

Positive Outcomes

- They were able to get a laryngoscope from emergency and managed the situation.
- The staffs were able to identify the mistake and accepted to follow the protocol.

Errors Encountered

- The staff in charge did not check the functioning of the equipment before handing it over to the doctor.
- Every shift, the functioning of equipment was not done.
- Proper assignment of special responsibility on equipment check was not done.
- The ward in charge should have ensured the working of equipment in the unit.
- Patient intubation was delayed leading to complications.

Lessons Learned

For nurse	For nurse educator	For nurse administrator
• Daily/every shift checking of critical equipment and drugs. • Clear assignment of duty (trolley, equipment, etc. checking) by incharge. • Cross checking by the incharge. • Ensure procedure readiness.	Train nurses on emergency readiness using simulation-based scenarios using such adverse events.	• To ensure availability of complete sealed crash cart at all the time. • Institute the checking of critical equipment, like laryngoscope, Defib, etc. in each shift. • Conduct audits by the nurse supervisor/incharge • Schedule rounds by the nursing supervisor to conduct random checks.

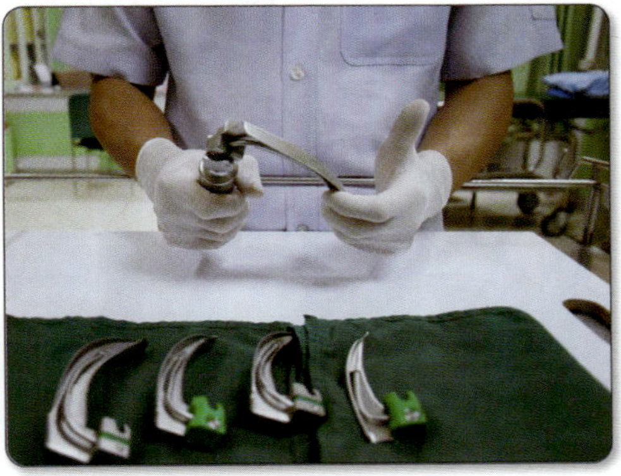

Figure 14 Laryngoscope

Event-Based Learning Summary

The critical incident highlights the paramount importance of complete and accurate communication during handovers in healthcare. When information is not conveyed thoroughly, errors can occur, potentially leading to severe consequences for the patient. In this case, a missing battery inside the laryngoscope caused a significant delay in a lifesaving procedure, leading to complications. The takeaway message is clear:

"Healthcare professionals must prioritize comprehensive and precise communication during handovers to ensure that critical details, such as equipment readiness, are conveyed accurately, thus safeguarding patient safety and well-being."

This incident also highlights the need for proper functionality of all critical life-saving equipment like the laryngoscope, defibrillator, oxygen cylinder by the assigned nurse before beginning of each shift.

There is no recovery from the harm that could happen to the patient if such equipment fail when they are needed the most.

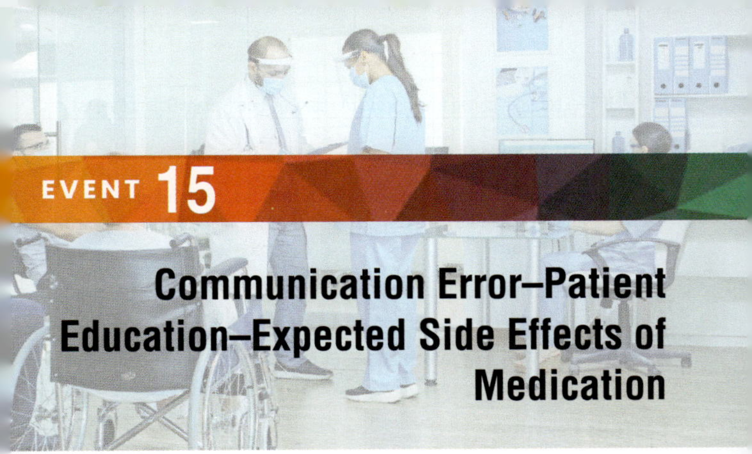

EVENT 15

Communication Error–Patient Education–Expected Side Effects of Medication

EVENT NO.	PSE/015/092022
IPSG RELATED TO	IPSG 2 – Improve Effective Communication

CASE STUDY DESCRIPTION

Mrs Rashmi, a 40-year-old patient was admitted on 01/02/2022 with complaints of increased menstrual bleeding, pale conjunctiva, weakness, fatigue, and tiredness. A gynecologist saw the patient, and some investigations were done. Hemoglobin (Hb) was 4.6 g/dL.

The doctor diagnosed metrorrhagia with severe anemia. The patient was treated with medical management. The patient's condition improved and was discharged on 10/02/2022. Rx: to control PV bleeding—Trapic 500 mg per oral TDS, 1-unit PRBC Blood transfusion and Ferric Carboxymaltose (FCM) transfusion done. Discharge advise included oral iron tablets to start after 7 days of discharge.

After 10 days, Mrs Rashmi got readmitted on 20/02/2022 with complaints of black tarry stools and fatigue.

On further communication with the patient and attendants, it was found that the nurses had not educated the patient about the expected effects FCM and oral Iron tablets and when to seek medical attention.

Positive Outcomes

- Nurses educated the patient about diet, hygiene, rest and exercise.
- The nurse explained warning signs of—PV bleeding, tachycardia, hypotension, etc.

Errors Encountered

- Inadequate education regarding side effects of oral iron tablets.
- Attendants were not informed about change in the stool color due to oral iron tablets.

Lessons Learned

For nurse	For nurse educator	For nurse administrator
• Ensure to educate patient on each drug that are being administered. • Ensure discharge education includes any expected side effects of the medications. • Use Teach-Back to ensure understanding.	Train nurses on discharge teaching checklist using various discharge scenarios.	• Develop SOP on discharge education. • Condition specific education handout can be made available in the hospital. • Important discharge information must be documented and counter signed by the companions and a copy maintained.

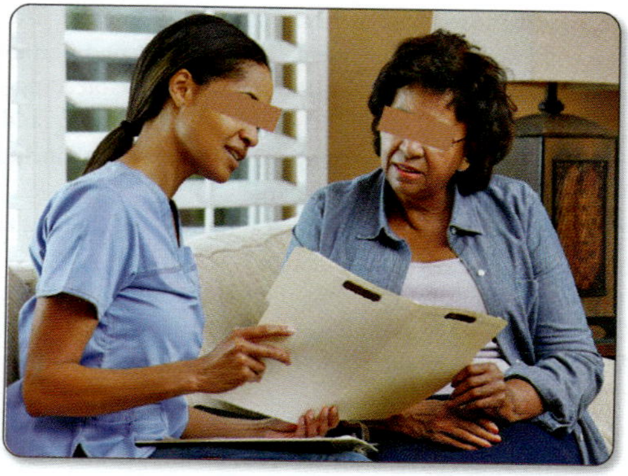

Figure 15 Nurse providing health education to patient

Event-Based Learning Summary

In healthcare, thorough patient education is pivotal for their well-being and comprehension of treatment. It is imperative to educate patients on both general care instructions and specific treatment details, including expected effects like changes in stool color. Equally important is extending this education to attendants or family members, ensuring everyone is informed. Moreover, the "Teach-Back" technique, where patients are encouraged to explain the information they have received, can confirm their understanding and reinforce effective communication. This comprehensive approach empowers patients and their caregivers, enabling them to actively participate in their care, recognize warning signs, and promptly seek medical assistance when necessary, ultimately enhancing patient safety and outcomes.

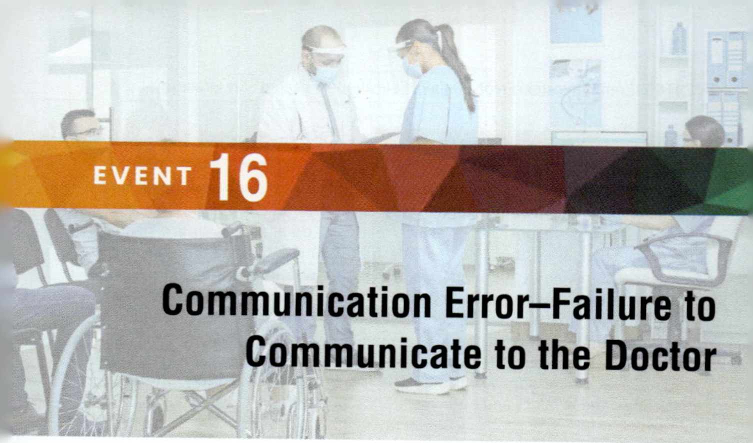

EVENT 16

Communication Error–Failure to Communicate to the Doctor

EVENT NO.	PSE/016/092022
IPSG RELATED TO	IPSG 2 – Improve Effective Communication

CASE STUDY DESCRIPTION

A 29-year-old female primi mother came to the antenatal clinic for a routine check-up on 04/01/2022. Vital signs were checked and recorded. The obstetrician had seen the patient and done USG and routine investigations. The obstetrician had diagnosed gestational diabetes mellitus (GDM), and the patient was medically managed with capillary blood glucose (CBG) charting. On the third day, the shift nurse failed to communicate high CBG findings to the doctor. Hence patient's insulin was not changed and the patient's CBG further increased. Later, the next shift duty nurse rechecked CBG, found the nurse's updates, informed the doctor and the patient's dose was titrated.

Positive Outcome

The nurses documented the CBG.

Errors Encountered

- Failed to communicate with the doctor.
- Failed to follow-up the patient care.

Lessons Learned

For nurse	For nurse educator	For nurse administrator
Critical alerts to be picked with due diligence and also to be escalated on real time.	• Train nurses on escalation matrix and critical alert. • Train nurses on consequences of high and low blood sugar. (hyper and hypoglycemia).	Design escalation matrix for the critical values and findings.

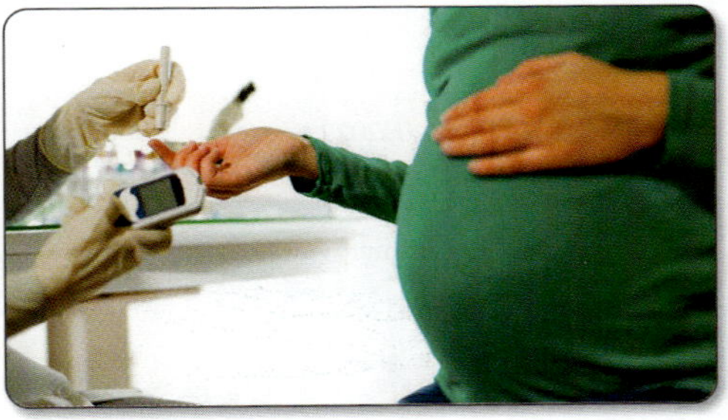

Figure 16 Pregnant woman with high capillary blood glucose

Event-Based Learning Summary

The event underscores the vital importance of effective communication in patient care. In this case, a communication breakdown led to delayed adjustment of a patient's insulin dose, resulting in high blood sugar levels. The Event-based Learning Summary is clear:

"Communication is a cornerstone of patient safety. Always prioritize timely and clear communication with the healthcare team, especially when it comes to critical patient information. In this case, high CBG findings should have been promptly conveyed to the doctor to ensure the patient's insulin was adjusted appropriately. Additionally, it is crucial to follow up on patient care to prevent lapses. By enhancing communication and vigilance in patient monitoring, we can provide safer and more effective care, ultimately benefiting our patients' well-being and outcomes."

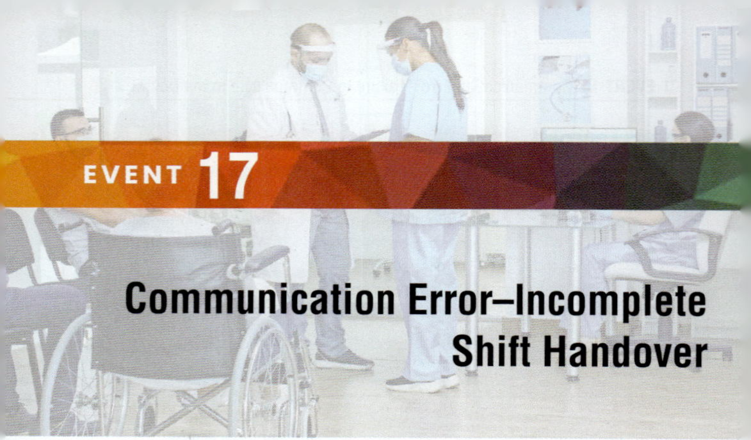

EVENT 17

Communication Error–Incomplete Shift Handover

EVENT NO.	PSE/017/092022
IPSG RELATED TO	IPSG 2 – Improve Effective Communication

CASE STUDY DESCRIPTION

Mrs Babita, a 46-year-old female, came to gynecology OPD on 20/12/2021 with complaints of irregular vaginal bleeding, weight loss, and lower abdominal pain. The gynecologist saw the patient and ordered for investigations, like PAP smear, CBC, USG and CT scan. CT scan showed an ovarian tumor. The patient had Hb of 6.5 mg/dL; hence, the doctor ordered 1 unit of PRBC. After the transfusion, a repeat Hb was ordered. At the end of the shift, the nurse took the blood sample and sent it to the lab. During the handing over, she forgot to communicate this to the next shift nurse. When the nurse prepared to collect the sample, the patient questioned that "Previous shift nurse had already taken the sample, then why are you taking the sample again?"

Positive Outcomes

- The previous shift nurse explained the purpose of the procedure (blood sample collection).
- The second shift nurse confirmed with lab, about the sample as claimed by the patient.
- Thus, the second prick and second sample was avoided.

Errors Encountered

- Incomplete communication during handing over, which could have resulted in 2nd prick for the patient.
- There was no documentation regarding the sample sent to the lab in the nurses' documentation.

Lessons Learned

For nurse	For nurse educator	For nurse administrator
• Handover communication is crucial during a shift change to maintain continuity of care and prevent errors. • Ensure it is documented as well. • Communication with patient before any procedure is crucial.	• Train nurses on shift endorsement and its importance with a role play. • Simulation-based and scenario-based training can be imparted to train nurses on the pitfalls of inadequate communication.	• Design structured template for the handing over process. • Ensure strong focus on the importance of communication to prevent patient harm.

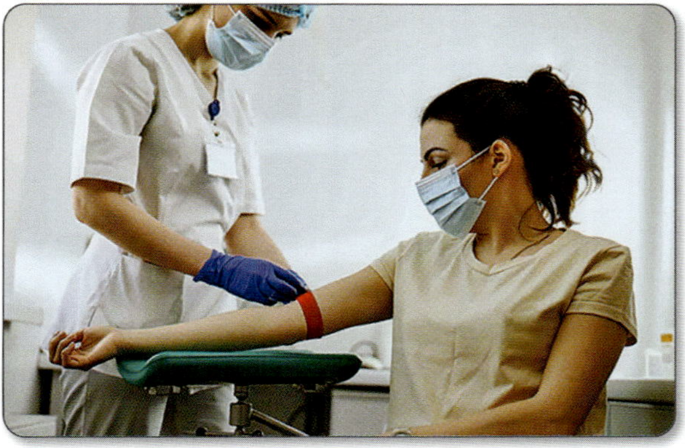

Figure 17 Nurse collecting blood sample

Event-Based Learning Summary

The scenario highlights the critical importance of effective communication during shift handovers. In this case, the oversight could have led to a second blood sample being collected from the patient, which is not ideal. The takeaway message for healthcare professionals, especially nurses, is as follows:

"Clear and thorough communication during shift handovers is essential to maintain patient safety and prevent unnecessary procedures. The incident underlines the need for diligent communication and documentation. When a patient's care involves procedures like blood sample collection, it is crucial to convey this information to the next shift, ensuring that everyone is on the same page. In this case, confirming with the laboratory was a prudent step, even when the patient verbalized her concern. By emphasizing proper handover communication and documentation, we can prevent misunderstandings unnecessary interventions, and ultimately enhance the quality of care we provide to our patients."

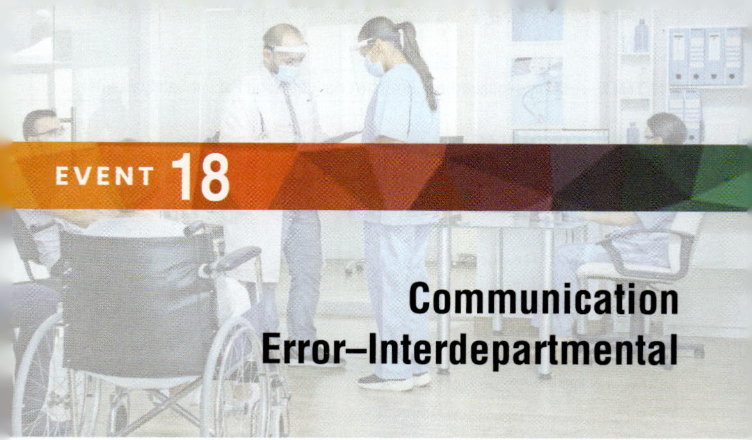

EVENT 18

Communication Error–Interdepartmental

EVENT NO.	PSE/018/092022
IPSG RELATED TO	IPSG 2 – Improve Effective Communication

CASE STUDY DESCRIPTION

The patient, Mahesh, was transferred to the plastic surgery ward from the OT after split skin grafting in his left lower limb. The immediate postoperative period was uneventful, and the postoperative orders included Inj. Heparin 5000 units in 500 mL of NS (8 drops/mt) for 2 days. The senior nurse didn't note the protocol (Heparin infusion for 5 days) and asked the doctor if she needs to continue on the 2nd postoperative day (POD).

He advised following the hospital protocol for heparin infusion. But the nurse stopped the Heparin infusion. The senior nurse received and documented the aPTT (40 seconds) value. In the evening the doctor came for rounds and found that the heparin was not given to the patient despite aPTT value being in the sub therapeutic range. He checked with the duty nurse and identified the communication error between the senior nurse and the assigned nurse. Hence the doctor reassessed the patient, and the heparin infusion was started again.

Positive Outcome

None.

Errors Encountered

- Patient's required therapy was interrupted.
  - The senior nurse did not refer the hospital protocol of Heparin for 5 days.
    - The nurse documented the aPTT value but did not communicate to the doctor, failing to note that this is the sub optimal value.

Lessons Learned

For nurse	For nurse educator	For nurse administrator
• Handover communication is a crucial transition of care to maintain continuity of care and prevent errors. • Ensure its documented as well. • Ensure no verbal order is taken. • Telephonic orders must be documented immediately and countersigned by the prescribing doctor as soon as possible. • Learn about anticoagulation and the related lab values.	• Train nurses on patient handover between the department and its importance with a role play. • Ensure to include verbal/telephonic order policy in the induction to ensure all new joinees know these protocols.	Create learning environment for all assigned nurses to know about all medications they administer to their patients (Quick Drug Reference books)

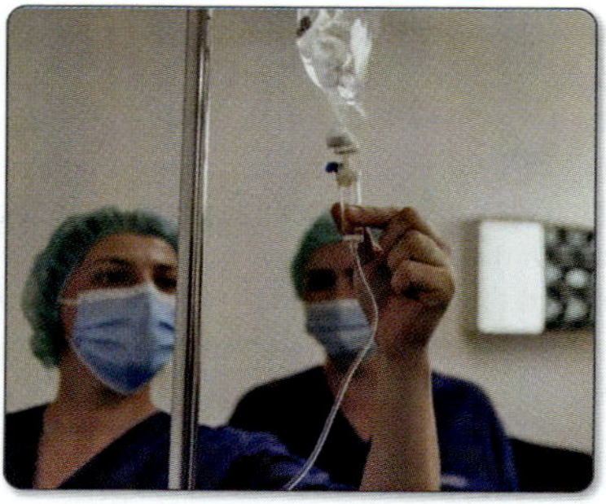

Figure 18 Communication between two nurses for heparin infusion

Event-Based Learning Summary

The event highlights the significance of effective interdepartmental communication within the healthcare system. In this case, a communication error led to a disruption in the patient's treatment plan. The takeaway message for healthcare professionals is as follows:

"Seamless interdepartmental communication is essential to ensure the continuity of patient care. It is imperative to not only initiate discussions about treatment plans, as seen when the senior nurse asked the doctor for clarification, but also to follow through by documenting critical information, such as laboratory values, and effectively communicate this data to the relevant medical professionals. This ensures that patient care remains consistent and uninterrupted. The incident emphasizes the importance of closing the loop in communication to prevent therapy disruptions and maintain the highest quality of care."

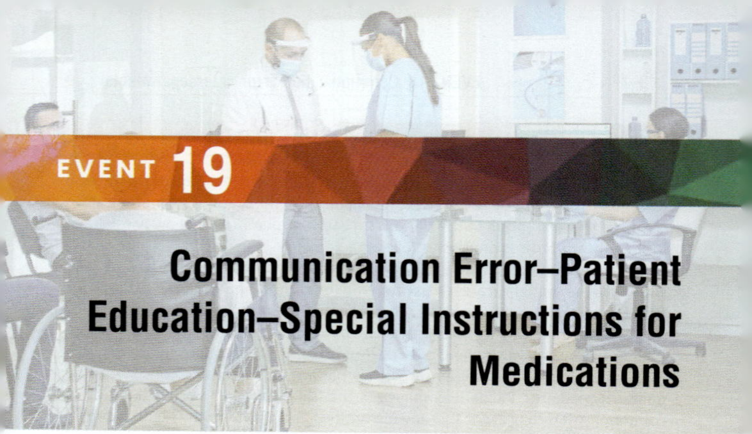

EVENT 19

Communication Error–Patient Education–Special Instructions for Medications

EVENT NO.	PSE/019/092022
IPSG RELATED TO	IPSG 2 – Improve Effective Communication

CASE STUDY DESCRIPTION

A 58-year-old male patient, a follow-up case of coronary bypass graft surgery, visited the cardiac OPD on the 34th postoperative day with chief complaints of sharp epigastric pain, dizziness, sweating, and feeling weakness. The attending physician assessed the patient and performed an emergency ECG monitoring and 2-D Echo, which were found to be within normal limits. Apparently the patient had taken Tab. Atorva 10 mg medication on empty stomach. It was figured out that the nurse had not explained the need for taking medicine after meals.

Positive Outcome

The nurse taught about when and how to obtain urgent care at discharge teaching.

Errors Encountered

- The patient was not educated to take medicines after meals.
- The nurse didn't follow the discharge teaching protocol.

Lessons Learned

For nurse	For nurse educator	For nurse administrator
• Make sure the patient is educated on each drug that are being administered. • Ensure discharge education.	Train nurses on discharge teaching checklist.	• SOP on discharge education. • Condition-specific education handout can be made available in the hospital. • Important discharge information must be documented and countersigned by the patient/attendant and a copy maintained. • Conduct random audits on discharge educations accuracy and completeness by using Teach-Back checklist.

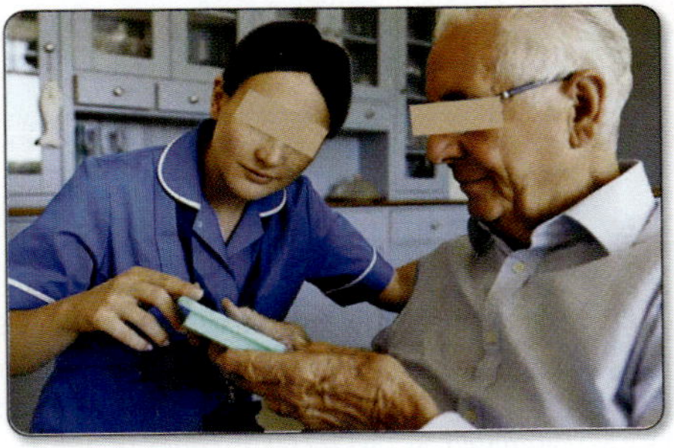

Figure 19 Nurse teaching patient for medication

Event-Based Learning Summary

This event emphasizes the critical role of patient education in healthcare. To ensure patients' safety and well-being, it is essential to communicate important instructions regarding their medications and care effectively. In this case, the nurse's initial teaching about when to seek urgent care at discharge was a positive step. However, the error occurred because the need for taking medication after meals was not adequately explained. The key takeaway message for healthcare professionals is as follows:

"Thorough patient education is a cornerstone of safe and effective healthcare. Beyond simply providing instructions, it is crucial to ensure that patients fully understand why, when, and how to follow these instructions. In this case, the oversight concerning medication administration highlighted the importance of clear and comprehensive patient education. It is imperative to go beyond providing information and confirm the patient's understanding to prevent medication errors and ensure their well-being throughout their treatment journey."

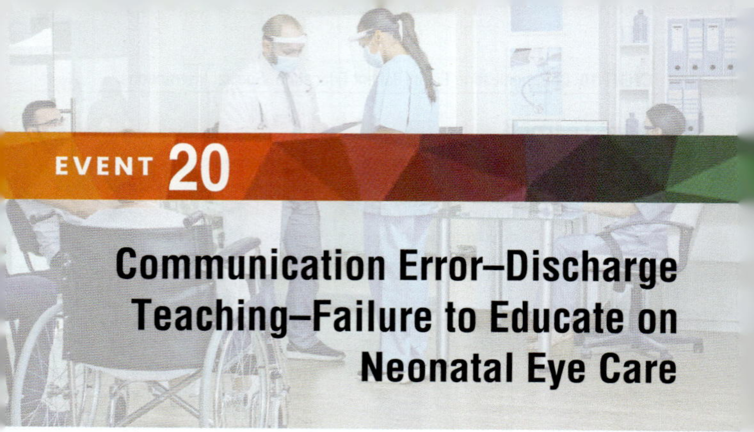

EVENT 20

Communication Error–Discharge Teaching–Failure to Educate on Neonatal Eye Care

EVENT NO.	PSE/020/092022
IPSG RELATED TO	IPSG 2 – Improve Effective Communication

CASE STUDY DESCRIPTION

A 27-year-old female primi mother delivered a live/term/male baby on 12/12/21. After a spontaneous vaginal delivery, she got discharged along with her baby after 5 days of delivery on 17/12/21.

The baby was readmitted on 28/12/21 with complaints of eye discharge, frequent crying, irritability, swelling, and redness over the eyes.

A pediatrician has seen the baby and diagnosed it as (ophthalmia neonatorum) neonatal conjunctivitis.

Positive Outcome

Nurse educated the mother about medication and immunization.

Errors Encountered

Nurses did not teach about eye care and hygiene and when to seek medical advice.

Lessons Learned

For nurse	For nurse educator	For nurse administrator
• Educate mothers/ parents and families about aspects of newborn care, including eye care, which could prevent the baby from getting admitted again. • Ensure discharge education. • Discharge information given must be countersigned by the patient and attendant.	• Train nurses on discharge teaching using checklist. • Train nurses on specialty specific patient education. • Train nurses on Teach Back policy.	• Developing education material on newborn care for parents to prevent such lapses. • Condition-specific education handout can be made available in the hospital. • Important discharge information must be documented and countersigned by the patient and attendant and a copy maintained.

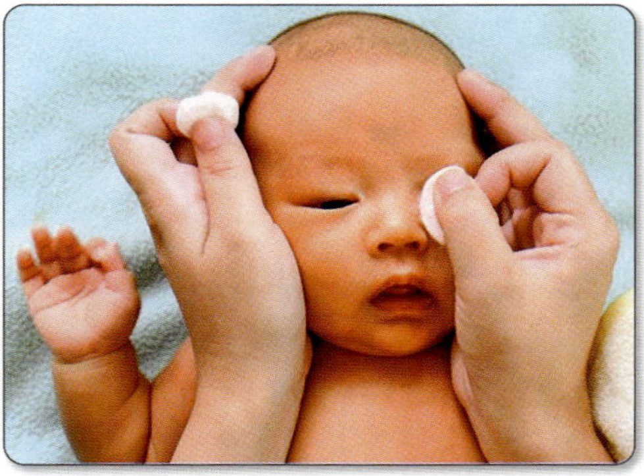

Figure 20 Nurse forgot to teach about eye care to mother

Event-Based Learning Summary

This case emphasizes the critical importance of comprehensive discharge teaching in healthcare. While the nurse did provide information about medication and immunization, the absence of education on basic eye care and hygiene, as well as when to seek medical advice, led to a significant issue. To ensure patient understanding, it is crucial to employ the "Teach-Back" method during discharge teaching. This approach encourages patients to explain the provided information, confirming their comprehension and empowering them to provide the best care for themselves and their newborns. By covering all relevant aspects of care and employing "Teach-Back" method, we can enhance patient knowledge and participation, ultimately contributing to better health outcomes.

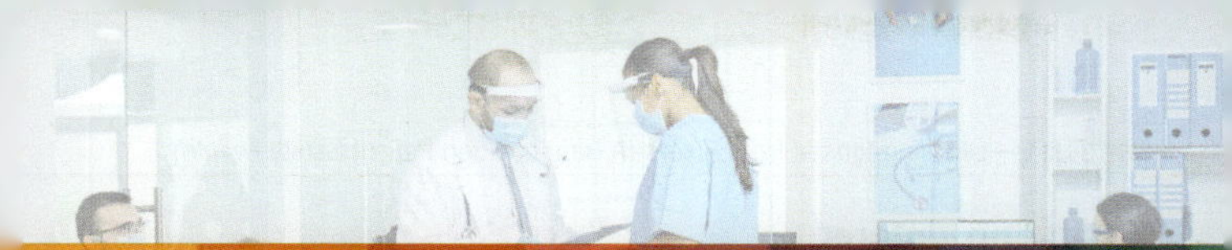

EVENT 21

Communication Error–Discharge Teaching–Failure to Teach About Febrile Seizures

EVENT NO.	PSE/021/092022
IPSG RELATED TO	IPSG 2 – Improve Effective Communication

CASE STUDY DESCRIPTION

A 4-month-old female child was admitted with complaints of increased body temperature, lethargy, and inability to suck.

The pediatrician examined the baby and diagnosed her with hyperthermia (temperature: 101°F). She was medically managed and discharged after three days.

After 12 days of discharge, the baby was readmitted with complaints of increased body temperature, abnormal eye movements, and jerky movement of extremities for 5 seconds. The pediatrician diagnosed the baby with febrile seizures.

Positive Outcomes

The parents were educated about:

- Medications
- Breastfeeding
- Hygiene
- Environmental safety

Errors Encountered

- Failed to teach about hyperthermia and its complications.
- Not educated about the tepid sponge.

Lessons Learned

For nurse	For nurse educator	For nurse administrator
• Educate parents on preventing febrile seizures in babies with high grade fever. • Use TEACH-BACK technique to confirm understanding of patient education.	• Train nurses on discharge teaching using a checklist. • Practice with role plays to train nurses TEACH-BACK technique.	• Condition-specific education handout can be made available in the hospital. • Implement audits on patient's discharge education.

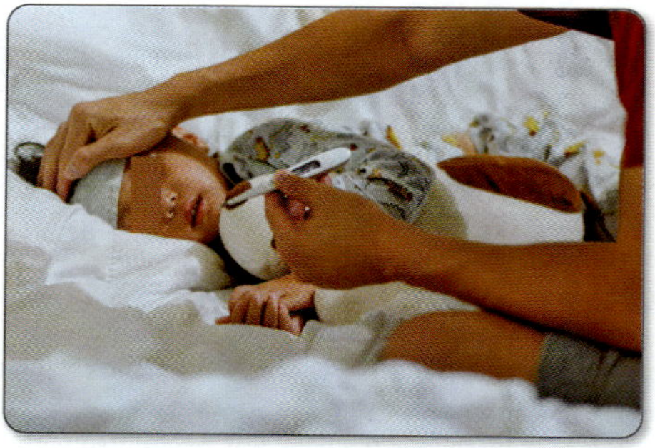

Figure 21 Tepid sponge

Event-Based Learning Summary

Effective discharge teaching is crucial to ensure the health and safety of pediatric patients. While the medical team did well in terms of medication management, breastfeeding support, hygiene, and environmental safety, there were notable gaps in education. Caregivers were not adequately informed about hyperthermia and its complications, and the valuable technique of tepid sponging was overlooked. To improve this, it is vital to educate caregivers thoroughly and employ the "TEACH-BACK" technique to confirm their understanding, ensuring they can confidently care for their child at home and prevent potential complications.

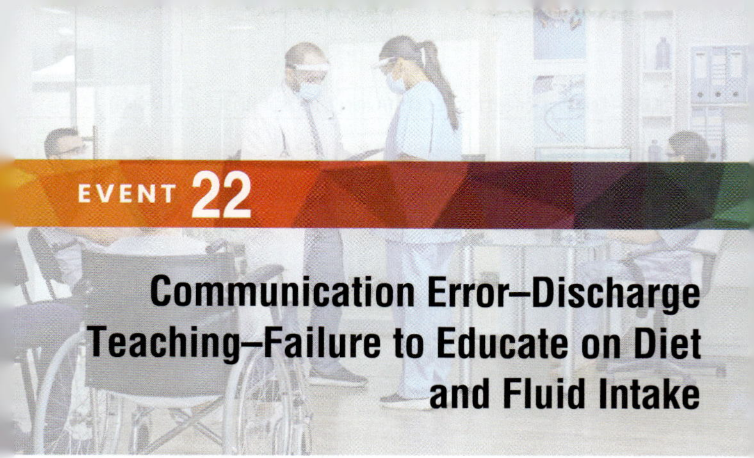

EVENT 22

Communication Error–Discharge Teaching–Failure to Educate on Diet and Fluid Intake

EVENT NO.	PSE/022/092022
IPSG RELATED TO	IPSG 2 – Improve Effective Communication

CASE STUDY DESCRIPTION

A 45-year-old female patient complained of heavy menstrual bleeding and white discharge per vagina.

The gynecologist examined the patient and performed PAP smear, CBC, and USG.

The patient was diagnosed with abnormal uterine bleeding (leiomyoma), and a Total Abdominal Hysterectomy was done. After 6 days, the patient got discharged.

After 8 days of discharge, the patient was re-admitted with complaints of abdominal distension, cramping, and constipation for three days. The patient was not informed regarding fluid balance and thought she would bleed more if she consumed more water.

Positive Outcome

The nurse explained postoperative care, such as postoperative exercises and medications.

Error Encountered

Nurses failed to educate regarding diet, adequate fluid intake, and the relationship between hydration and constipation.

Lessons Learned

For nurse	For nurse educator	For nurse administrator
• Effective and relevant discharge teaching is essential to enable the patient to care for themself following discharge, preventing complications. • Use TEACH-BACK technique to confirm understanding of patient education.	• Train nurses on discharge teaching checklist. • Practice with role plays to train nurses TEACH-BACK technique.	• Condition specific education handout can be made available in the hospital. • Implement audits on patient's discharge education.

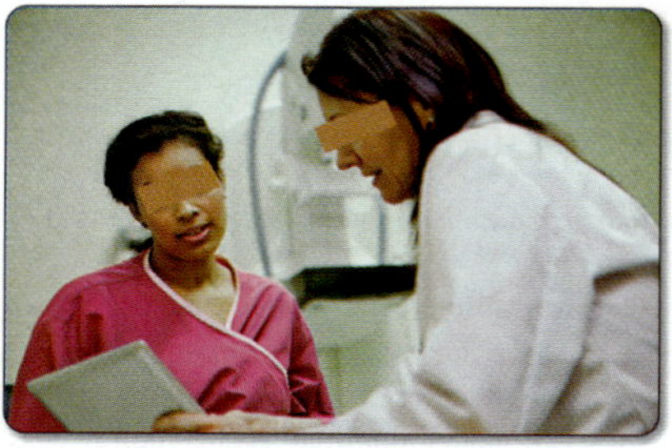

Figure 22 Nurse giving education to patient after abdominal hysterectomy

Event-Based Learning Summary

Comprehensive discharge teaching is essential in postoperative care, as highlighted in this case. While the nurse successfully explained postoperative care aspects like exercises and medication, there was a notable failure to educate the patient about her diet and the importance of adequate fluid intake. This led to a misconception where the patient believed that drinking more water would increase bleeding, resulting in abdominal issues and constipation. The take-home message is clear; it is crucial to provide patients with comprehensive postoperative instructions, including dietary and hydration guidance, to avoid misconceptions and complications, fostering a smoother recovery process. Clear and thorough communication is key to preventing such issues. Using TEACH-BACK technique can ensure patient understanding.

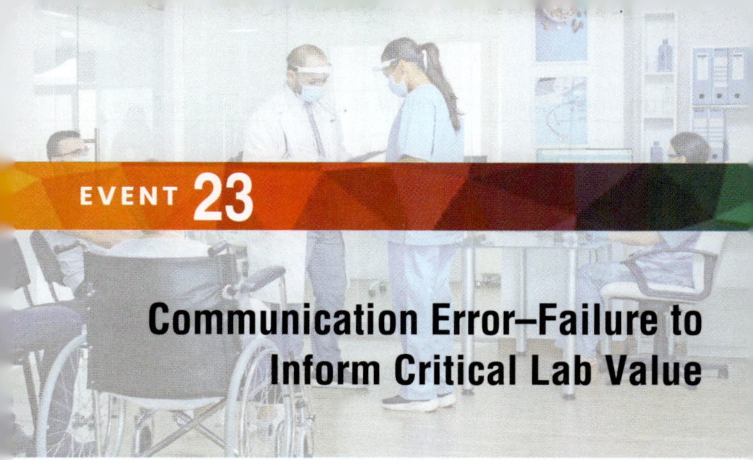

EVENT 23

Communication Error–Failure to Inform Critical Lab Value

EVENT NO.	PSE/023/092022
IPSG RELATED TO	IPSG 2 – Improve Effective Communication

CASE STUDY DESCRIPTION

A 22-year-old female was admitted to the medical ward with fever. On admission, the basic investigations and fever profile was sent. The fever profile was negative. On the third day, around 1.20 am, she complained of abdominal pain and decreased urine output. The nurse informed the duty doctor. She examined the patient and the Foley's catheter was inserted. Nearly 300 mL of urine was drained with gross hematuria. The duty doctor viewed the case sheet and investigation chart and found that the patient had thrombocytopenia with a platelet count of 10,000, which was a critical lab value, which was not communicated to the doctor as per the hospital policy. The nursing staff received the critical lab alert around 9 pm but failed to communicate to the physician. Later the patient was shifted to the high-dependency unit and treated for thrombocytopenia.

Positive Outcomes

- The staff nurse informed the doctor about abdominal pain without any delay.
- The team had shifted the patient to a high dependency unit for further management.

Errors Encountered

- The critical lab value was not informed to the doctor.
- The critical lab value was not documented in the critical alert register.

Lessons Learned

For nurse	For nurse educator	For nurse administrator
Critical alerts to be escalated on real time.	• Train nurses on escalation matrix and critical alerts. • Train nurses on rationale for critical lab alerts and its significance on patient's safety.	• Design escalation matrix for the critical values and findings and the documentation template. • Implement audits for compliance to the protocol on critical lab alerts.

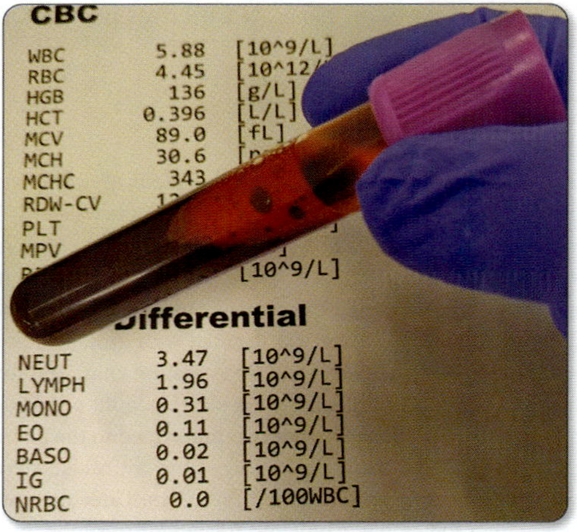

Figure 23 Lab values

Event-Based Learning Summary

While the prompt response to abdominal pain and the patient's transfer to a high-dependency unit were positive aspects, the failure to communicate and document the critical lab value of thrombocytopenia (platelet count of 10,000) was a critical oversight. Healthcare providers must strictly adhere to hospital policies for managing such situations, emphasizing the need for immediate action based on these values. Clear and comprehensive communication, both about lab values and changes in the patient's condition, is paramount in ensuring effective and timely patient care.

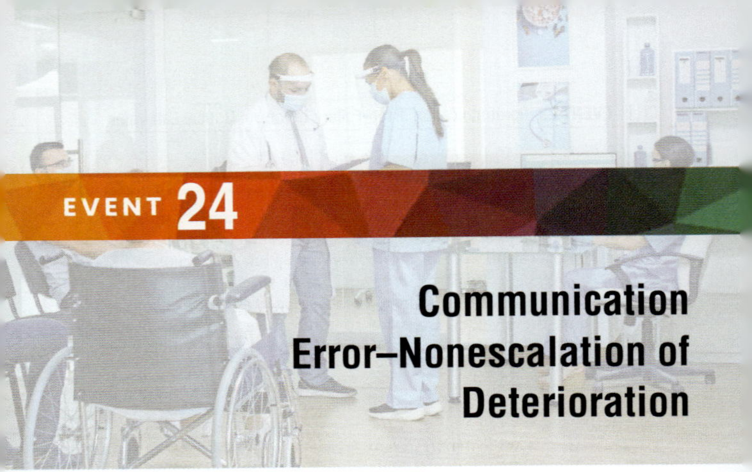

EVENT 24

Communication Error–Nonescalation of Deterioration

EVENT NO.	PSE/024/092022
IPSG RELATED TO	IPSG 2 – Improve Effective Communication

CASE STUDY DESCRIPTION

A 60-year-old female patient was admitted with complaints of abdominal pain and vomiting. The patient had history of multiple abdominal surgeries including a gastric bypass surgery. The patient was examined and admitted for rehydration with IV fluids. The doctor also advised for bowel rest with minimal food intake. On the third day the patient started vomiting multiple times. The on-duty doctor referred her to the treating surgeon who has done the gastric bypass surgery. The patient continue to vomit in the night and also had tan colored emesis but the nurse did not inform anyone even though she has documented it. The next day patient's family took the patient to another hospital as they were not satisfied with the treatment. It was found that the patient had aspirated.

Positive Outcome

None.

Errors Encountered

- The on-duty nurse failed to communicate the patient's condition to the consultant.

- Nurses' note was not specific and clear.
- The nurses failed to observe criticality of tan colored emesis.

Lessons Learned

For nurse	For nurse educator	For nurse administrator
• Critical patient condition must be observed and escalated without any delay. • Nurses must inform even minor changes in the patient's conditions to their seniors or doctors.	• Provide comprehensive training on communication protocols, patient monitoring, and the importance of reporting changes in a patient's condition. • Practice such scenarios to train nurses on the fatal outcomes that can occur if nurses fail to observe and escalate deteriorating patient's condition on time.	• Implement clear communication protocols. • Create a culture that encourages and supports reporting. This includes recognizing and rewarding nurses who report changes in a patient's condition promptly. • Provide safe space for nurses to report concerns without fear of retaliation. • Schedule and conduct regular audits.

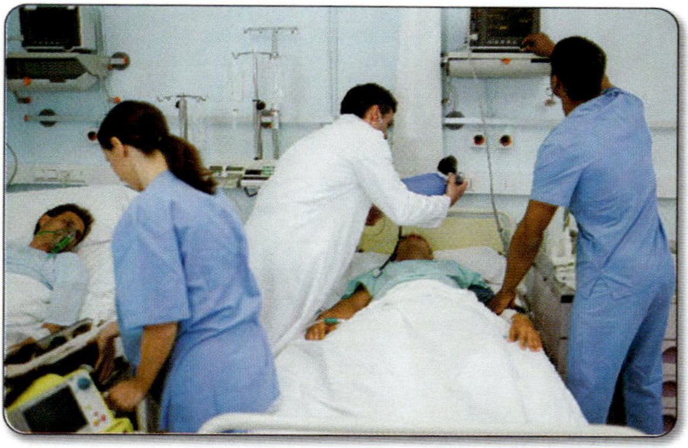

Figure 24 Nurses escalate the critical values to consultant and prompt action taken

Event-Based Learning Summary

This case underscores the crucial need for clear communication and detailed documentation in patient care. Inadequate reporting of a patient's deteriorating condition can have serious consequences. Additionally, it is essential to consider a patient's medical history, especially if they have a surgical history, and consult the relevant specialists promptly to prevent potential complications. These actions are fundamental in ensuring patient safety and timely intervention when needed. Nurse's diligence and timely communication play a pivotal role in providing quality care and preventing adverse outcomes.

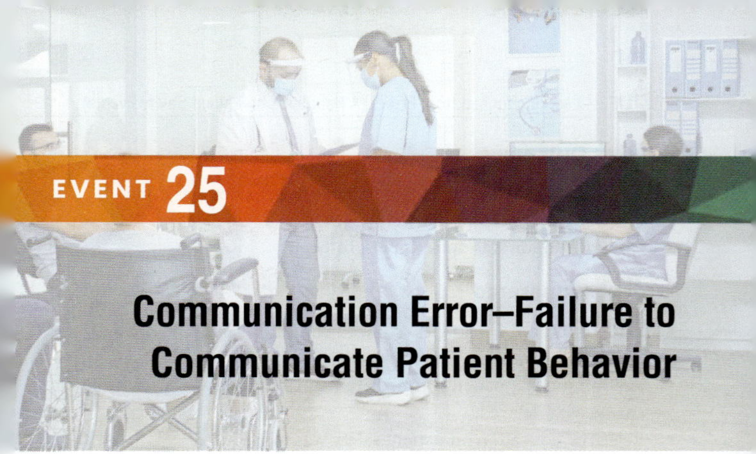

EVENT 25

Communication Error–Failure to Communicate Patient Behavior

EVENT NO.	PSE/025/092022
IPSG RELATED TO	IPSG 2 – Improve Effective Communication

CASE STUDY DESCRIPTION

The nurses must do the standard checks and observations for all the invasive lines and tubes, documents and update the records at every shift. A 73-year-old male patient was admitted with disorientation, agitated behavior and confused state of mind. The patient was restrained during the ICU stay. The patient was shifted to the floor when the agitation had settled. But some confusion was still prevailing. During the night shift the patient got agitated and could not be controlled by the assigned nurse and the relative. After immediate escalation, the duty doctor collaborated with the primary consultant and neurologist, who advised a sedative to be administered to the patient, STAT. Assigned nurse was preparing the drug near the nurse's station.

Meanwhile, the patient got out of the bed and started moving toward the washroom with the relative by his side. When the nurse entered the room, the patient had already pulled out his inflated foley's catheter causing him to bleed, with severe pain, and dribbling urine. On-Call urologist was paged, who examined the patient, and planned for scope-guided catheterization the next day.

Positive Outcomes

- Immediate escalation of patient change in behavior was done.
- Line reconciliation was done as per SOPs.
- Documentation was done as per protocol.

Errors Encountered

- Understanding a patient's clinical condition and anticipating the threats were missed.
- Restraining the patient immediately during observation of behavior change was delayed.
- Relatives' education on patient safety was inadequate.
- Anticipatory SOS orders for agitation were not in place.

Lessons Learned

For nurse	For nurse educator	For nurse administrator
• To be vigilant for anticipated threats while observing the patient. • To remain prepared for SOS orders. • Escalate the condition of the patient to the senior nurse/in-charge whenever the patient condition changes or becomes unmanageable.	• Staff education regarding managing the agitated patient and reaching out for immediate support from the senior staff. • Focus on training and retraining. • Use case studies and simulations to teach nurses to troubleshoot common problems. • Provide hands-on training where they can learn troubleshooting skills with real equipment and devices. • Emphasise using critical thinking. Encourage nurses to use their knowledge to come up with solutions.	• Acuity-based staffing can be implemented. • Induction training can be more scenario-based. • Having open discussions with the staff involved in the event can facilitate self-reflection and learning.

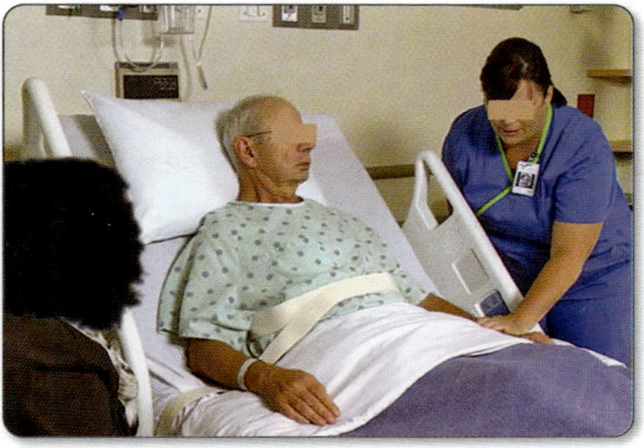

Figure 25 Nurse restraining the patient immediately when sudden behavior changes observed

Event-Based Learning Summary

The critical lesson from this case is the need for healthcare providers to fully grasp a patient's clinical condition and anticipate potential risks. Quick escalation during a change in a patient's behavior is essential. Moreover, clear "SOS" emergency protocols must be in place, especially for night-time scenarios when responses can be delayed. Equally vital is educating patients' families on patient safety to help manage situations and prevent harm. Adhering to established procedures, providing clear documentation, and ensuring all team members are aware of these protocols are vital in maintaining patient safety.

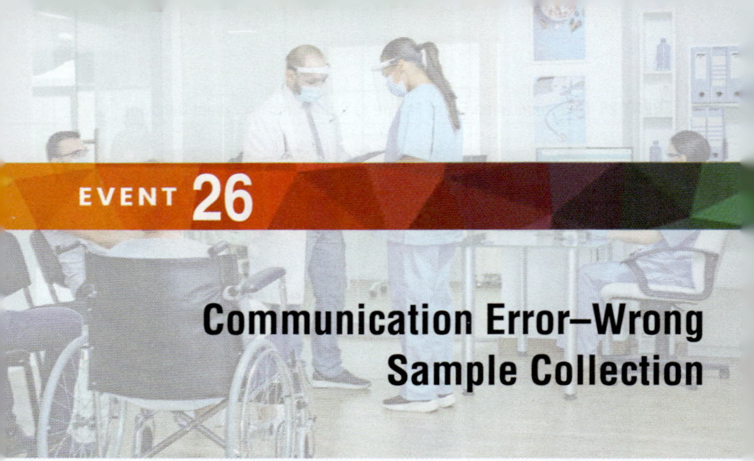

EVENT 26

Communication Error–Wrong Sample Collection

EVENT NO.	PSE/026/092022
IPSG RELATED TO	IPSG 2 – Improve Effective Communication

CASE STUDY DESCRIPTION

Mrs Swati was admitted to the medical ward with fever for evaluation. A set of investigations were ordered for the patient and samples dispatched to the laboratory. After the prescribed timeline there were no investigation reports available for the patient. It was found that the samples sent were of another patient who had a similar name in the ward. Issue was reported and samples were taken and sent to the laboratory for the correct patient.

Positive Outcomes

- Proper follow-up was done to get the laboratory results.
- The error was identified on time.
- Wrong diagnosis and treatment were prevented.
- Specimens were sent for the right patient after discovering the error.

Errors Encountered

- Proper identification of patients was not done.
- Unnecessary investigation, and pain for the patient who was wrongly identified.
- Delay to diagnose and treat the correct patient.

Lessons Learned

For nurse	For nurse educator	For nurse administrator
• Verify the patient's identification by asking the patient to state his/her name. • To use two patient identifiers during all the procedures by matching the information on the patient file with that of the patient's ID band. • Proceed with the sample collection only after the above two steps. • Keep in mind that there could be patients who have similar names (Spell-Alike_Sound-Alike). • Label the sample containers/ vacutainers after collecting the sample immediately. • Collect one patient sample at one time. Take articles required for that patient only. • Get another nurse to verify the order and samples.	• Train nurses on patient identification with reference to specimen collection. • In the training sessions, stress on the importance of labeling patient samples accurately and clearly. Explain the potential consequences of sample mixing and emphasize the need for vigilance and attention to detail. • Use case studies and scenarios to help trainees understand the risks associated with sample mixing and how to prevent it. • Use visual aids such as videos to help trainees understand the steps involved in sample collection and labeling. • Provide feedback and coaching to nurses to help them improve their skills and avoid errors. • Emphasize mistakes that can happen when patients are not identified correctly. • Enforce the need to involve the patient in the identification process and match the name and UHID in the patient record with that of the info on the ID band.	• SOP on specimen collection to have steps on patient identification. • Barcoding technology and use of electronic health records can be used to ensure that samples are accurately labeled and tracked throughout the testing process. • Use visual cues, such as color-coded labels or signage, to help staff members differentiate between samples from different patients. This can help reduce the risk of mix-ups and improve accuracy. • Plan and conduct audits to understand the compliance to the SOPs. • Ensure a process of identifying situations when patients with similar name are admitted to the same ward they are assigned to different nurses. • Such a situation can be flagged off in the hospital information system. • Alert notes can be placed on both patient's files.

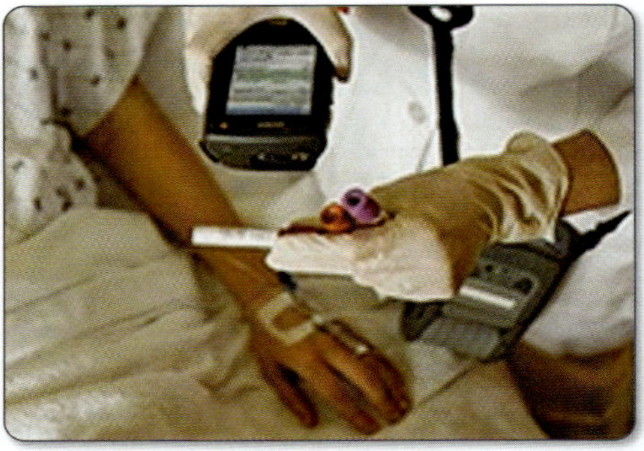

Figure 26 Positive patient identification during blood sampling

Event-Based Learning Summary

This case underscores the vital importance of proactive patient communication during sample collection. Ensuring patients are not only correctly identified but also informed about the tests being conducted can be a powerful preventive measure. Involving patients in this process could have averted the mix-up by allowing them to actively confirm their identity and understand the purpose of the tests. Such engagement empowers patients, minimizes the risk of sample errors, and promotes patient safety by fostering a cooperative approach between healthcare providers and patients they are caring for.

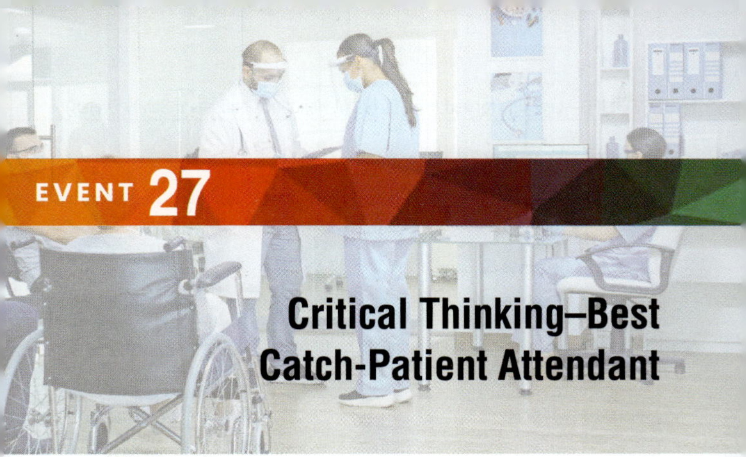

EVENT 27

Critical Thinking–Best Catch-Patient Attendant

EVENT NO.	PSE/027/092022
IPSG RELATED TO	None

CASE STUDY DESCRIPTION

A second-year BSc nursing student was assigned along with the staff nurse to a 65-year-old male patient who had undergone diabetic foot wound debridement in the general surgical ward. At 8:15 am, asking the patient for his breakfast, the patient told that he was waiting for his attendant to bring breakfast from outside but still has not returned. The patient requested the student to search for his attendant. Two student nurses searched everywhere in and around the ward. They waited half an hour for the attendant, thinking he must have gone out for something. One student thought of checking the bathrooms. He found one bathroom that was locked from inside and tried to call that person out. Since he did not get any response, the student nurse reported this incident to the ward in-charge and other staff. With their help, another student jumped into the restroom through the window and opened the door. The victim was the patient's attendant, and he was unresponsive. Immediate CPR was initiated but unfortunately the attendant could not be revived.

Positive Outcome

The student nurse had the presence of mind to check the bathrooms.

Errors Encountered

If the shift endorsement had been done at the bedside, the attendant's absence probably would have been identified earlier.

Lessons Learned

For nurse	For nurse educator	For nurse administrator
Endorsement to be done at the bedside. Ward rounds should include a tour of all areas of the unit.	Training on bedside rounds.	To ensure in-charge of the department covers all the areas in the ward during the rounds to pick such unfortunate event.

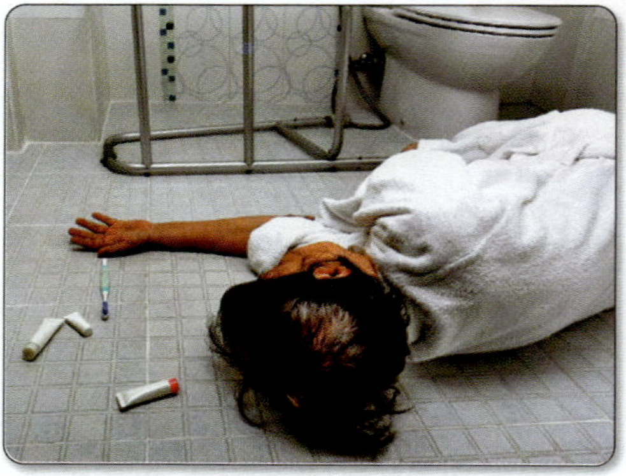

Figure 27 Patient's relative found dead in bathroom

Event-Based Learning Summary

This case highlights the importance of proactive patient-centered care. The student nurse's quick thinking and teamwork were commendable, but a more patient-centered approach to shift endorsements might have identified the attendant's absence earlier. Routine ward rounds, including restrooms, by healthcare staff, housekeeping, and security personnel, can help uncover unusual events and prevent tragic outcomes like the one in this incident.

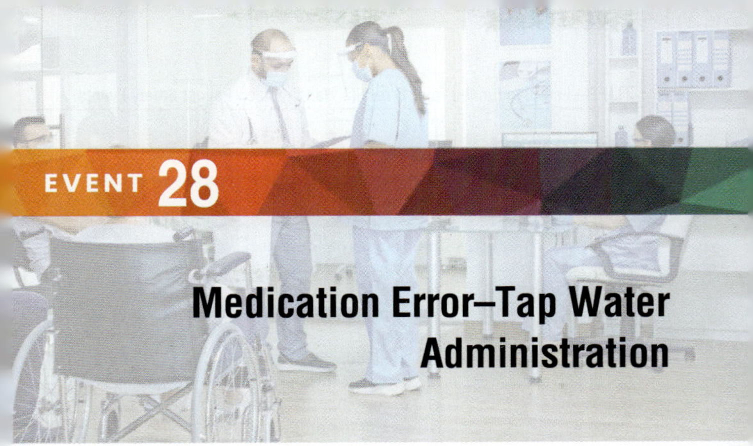

EVENT 28

Medication Error–Tap Water Administration

EVENT NO.	PSE/0028/092022
IPSG RELATED TO	None

CASE STUDY DESCRIPTION

A 40-year-old man was admitted for abdominal pain. At the time of medication administration, Inj. Voveran's ampule was dropped accidentally from the nurse and was broken. She got nervous; immediately came to the medication room, not knowing how to handle the situation, and loaded tap water and administered it to the patient. The next day patient started with a high-grade fever and had to be started on antibiotics.

Positive Outcome

Fortunately, the patient did not have fatal consequences from the action.

Errors Encountered

- The nurse failed to report.
- The nurse did something that should never have been done, amounting to malpractice.

Lessons Learned

For nurse	For nurse educator	For nurse administrator
• Report any occurrences to the seniors in the department. • Seek help when in doubt. • Document and report the incident. • Unethical practices should not be attempted on the patients.	• Train nurses on incident reporting process and reiterate the outcome and impact by building in confidence. • Provide feedback regarding the incident and ensure that the nurse is aware of the proper techniques for handling ampules to prevent them from breaking in the future. • The nurse educator can discuss common accidents that can happen and informing seniors for further guidance. • Emphasize the point that hiding accidents will not help anyone, rather reporting will help to learn how to prevent such accidents.	• Incorporate measures to encourage reporting culture in the department. • Rewarding and recognizing self reporting of accidents and mistakes can facilitate creating a safe environment. This will also prevent nurses from hiding accidents and mistakes.

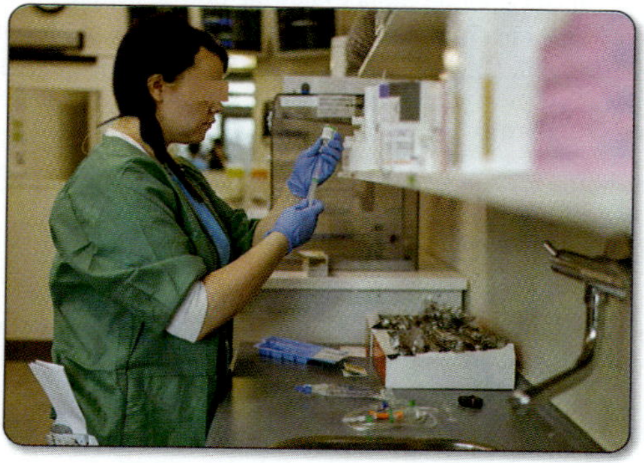

Figure 28 Nurse ensures safety while preparing the medication

Event-Based Learning Summary

The key takeaway from this incident is the critical need for nurses to remain composed in high-stress situations, prioritizing patient safety above all else. Errors can and do occur, but the fear of making a mistake should never compromise patient's well-being. Instead, healthcare professionals must have the courage to speak up and seek guidance or assistance when they encounter difficulties, ensuring they adhere to established protocols and provide the safest possible care. In the event of an error, timely reporting and collaboration with the healthcare team are vital to prevent potential harm and uphold patient safety as the utmost priority.

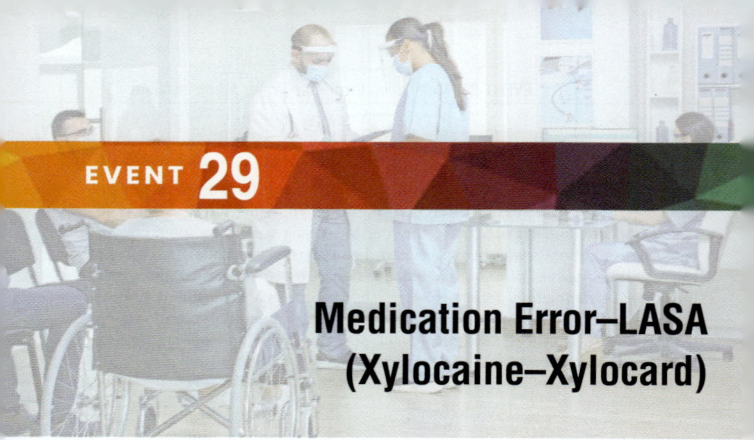

EVENT 29

Medication Error–LASA (Xylocaine–Xylocard)

EVENT NO.	PSE/029/092022
IPSG RELATED TO	IPSG 3 – Improve the Safety of High-Alert Medications

CASE STUDY DESCRIPTION

For a patient posted for surgery, there was a preoperative order to give Inj. Xylocaine test dose before shifting to OT. The staff nurse administered Inj. Xylocard (0.1 mL Intradermal), as the drug label, indicates "**Lignocaine Hydrochloride Injection**" for both drugs. It was found when the nurse gave the remaining drug to the OT staff nurse. Immediately it was escalated to the anesthetist; the patient's cardiac parameters were monitored, and the test dose was repeated with Inj. Xylocaine, and the surgery was rescheduled.

Positive Outcomes

- The staff nurse (ward) showed the vial to OT nurse and conveyed that this was the drug she had administered.
- The OT In-charge noticed it, and immediately the anesthetist was informed, and monitoring was done.
- The team handled the event without panicking the patient.

Errors Encountered

- The ward nurse didn't follow the LASA drug policy.
- Both the drugs were stored in the same cupboard rack.
- The look-alike sound-alike alert sticker was not present on the drug.
- The nurse who administered the drug should have read the drug label thrice, by which she would have probably realized the difference.

Lessons Learned

For nurse	For nurse educator	For nurse administrator
• To double verify medications before administration. • Be aware of LASA drugs policy and be familiar with the LASA drugs in the units.	• Train nurses on medication administration process. • Educate on list of high alert LASA medicine and related protocol.	• SOP and adherence to LASA and high alert medications to be in place. • Implement periodic audit to ensure safe practices are in place.

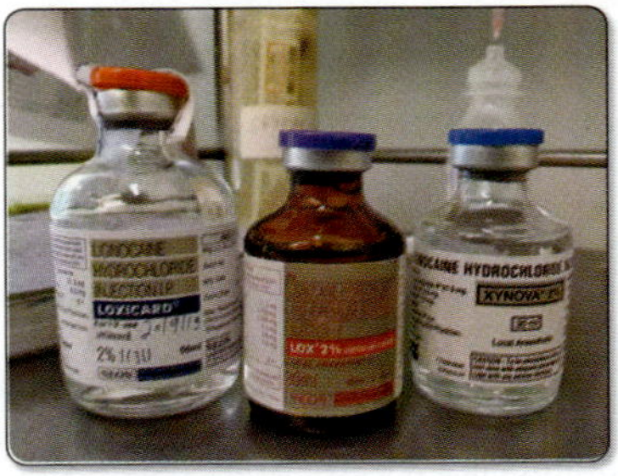

Figure 29 Difference between Inj. Xylocard and Inj. Xylocaine

Event-Based Learning Summary

This case underscores the critical need for healthcare professionals to follow Look-alike Sound-alike (LASA) drug policies diligently, especially in scenarios involving drugs with similar names. Effective communication and swift error escalation are vital in mitigating potential harm to patients. Additionally, it highlights the significance of personal accountability and the responsibility to double-check drug labels thoroughly to ensure patient safety. Clear labeling and proper drug storage are key elements in preventing such errors and upholding the highest standards of patient care.

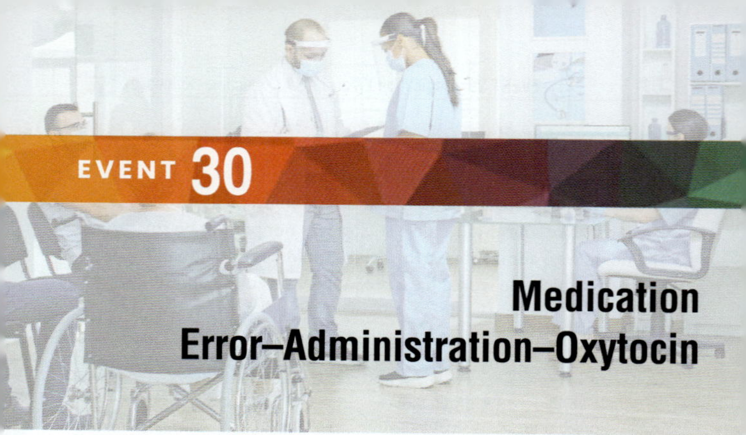

EVENT 30

Medication Error–Administration–Oxytocin

EVENT NO.	PSE/030/092022
IPSG RELATED TO	None

CASE STUDY DESCRIPTION

A full-term primi-para was posted for emergency cesarean section (CS) because of prolonged labor with fetal distress. The nurse assigned to the patient did all preparations for CS as per the checklist, and the patient was transferred to OT with normal saline on flow at the rate of 4 drops/mL. The OT nurse received the patient, and the anesthetist flushed the IV fluid rapidly as he wanted to start a new one as a routine procedure. Meanwhile, the OT nurse identified that the FHR was shooting up above 160, and the patient had rapid, muscular contractions. Immediately, the IV infusion was stopped, and on reading the transfer notes, oxytocin 5 units were added to the fluid, which caused rapid contraction upon increasing the flow. The nurse had written the transfer notes, but she had neither given an oral report nor labeled the IV bottle.

Positive Outcomes

- The nurse did all preparations as per the checklist before transfer.
- Wrote transfer notes appropriately.

Errors Encountered

- The intravenous fluid was not labeled regarding the additive drug; oxytocin.
- The OT nurse had neither received the oral report nor checked the transfer notes.
- The protocol for stopping the oxytocin infusion once the patient was posted for a cesarean section was not followed.

Lessons Learned

For nurse	For nurse educator	For nurse administrator
• Ensure that all the infusion are labeled with type of fluid and additives. • Ensure clear communication while handing over the patient and follow standing protocols on preparing patients for CS.	• Educate nurses on infusion practices and handing over process. • Ensure the nurses assigned to specialty areas are oriented to the departmental protocols, especially high-alert medications.	• Availability of ready infusion labels in the department. • Handing over documentation template for preoperative and postoperative. • Implement regular audits on safe handling of high-alert medications.

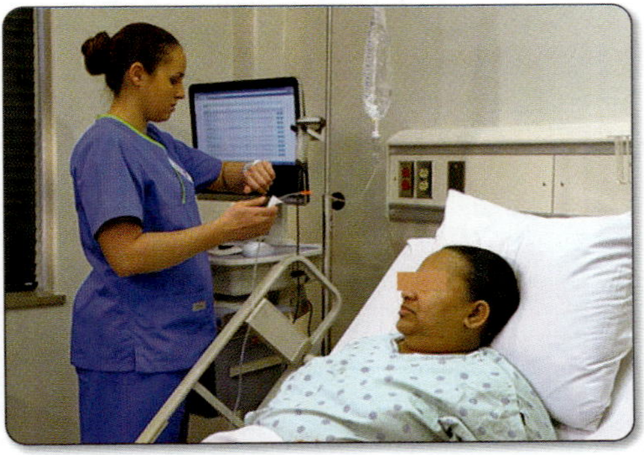

Figure 30 Nurse ensures the infusion is labeled and going on appropriate rate

Event-Based Learning Summary

This case highlights the pivotal role nurses play in medication safety. While the nurse diligently prepared the patient for a Cesarean Section and provided written transfer notes, crucial errors occurred. Failure to label the intravenous fluid regarding the high-alert additive drug, inadequate communication between nursing teams and non-compliance with protocols led to complications. Nurses should ensure patient safety, emphasize the significance of clear communication, adhere to established procedures, and diligent labeling in medication administration to prevent errors that may compromise patient's well-being.

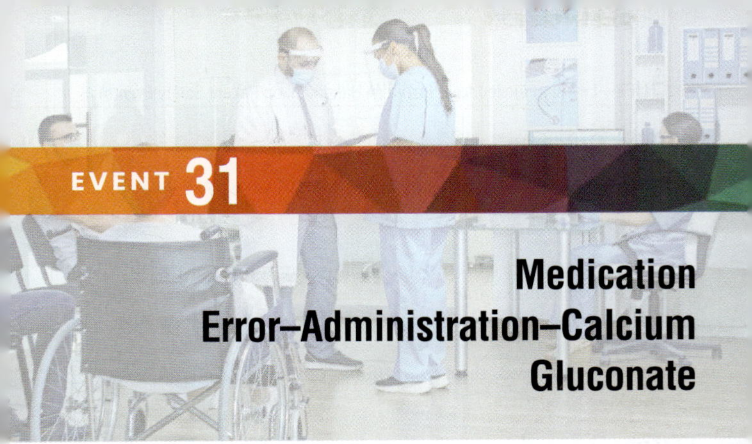

EVENT 31

Medication Error–Administration–Calcium Gluconate

EVENT NO.	PSE/031/092022
IPSG RELATED TO	IPSG 3 – Safe Handling of High-Risk Medication

CASE STUDY DESCRIPTION

A newborn female baby was admitted to neonatal intensive care unit (NICU) after birth with a Patent Ductus Arteriosus (PDA). During her stay in the NICU, she was on nil by mouth and on IV fluids, with continuous monitoring of heart rate, respiratory rate, BP, and SpO_2. The night duty staff nurse handed over to the morning duty staff. While handing over, she mentioned that medication Calcium Gluconate 0.1 mL diluted in 10 mL of normal saline to be given over 20 minutes. There were two syringes loaded and kept in the bedside locker. One was the diluted Calcium Gluconate, and another with the concentrated one. The night nurse mislabeled the syringes by mistake. As the handover was over, the morning staff gave the labeled medicine on the syringe pump, which was undiluted. After a few minutes, the monitor started beeping an alarm, showing a heart rate of zero. The morning staff thought the probe might have slipped out, and she tried to fix it, but it was zero again; then she thought it might be the error of the investigation, and her eyes went to the baby side too. She found the inactive baby and shouted for help. The intensivist on duty heard the alarm, noticed the zero heart rate and activated the Code Blue and at the same time the IV Calcium Gluconate was stopped. The baby could be revived.

Positive Outcome

Prompt activation of Code Blue by the intensivist could save the baby.

Errors Encountered

- The assigned nurse administered the infusion which was prepared and labeled by another nurse.
- The morning staff did not seek clarification as to why two syringes were loaded.
- The nurse wasted time confirming probe placement instead of checking the patient.

Lessons Learned

For nurse	For nurse educator	For nurse administrator
• Never administer any medication prepared and labeled by another nurse, unless it is prepared in your presence. • Calcium Gluconate is a high-risk medication, therefore always have one more nurse to counter check. • During handover, nurses must question each other in case of any doubts.	Appropriate and efficient training and supervision of critical care staff are essential to ensure nurses follow safe medication administration practices to prevent patient harm.	• Privileging of nurses on medication administration is mandatory. • Double check mandate by two nurses for high risks medications to be included in nursing SOP. • Use such scenarios during training. • Appropriate corrective and preventive actions, including process review and modifications following the RCA of errors, can prevent future mistakes.

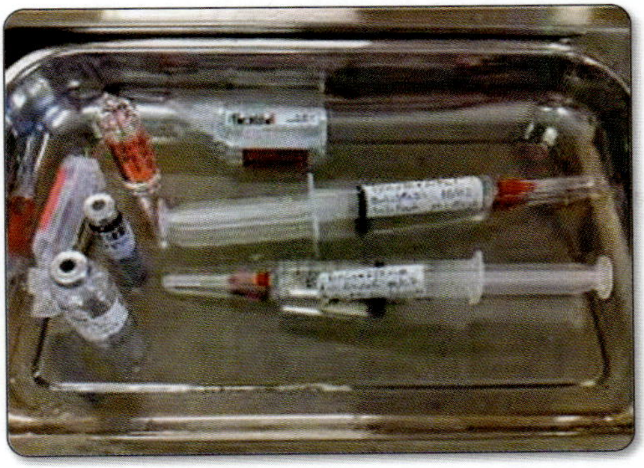

Figure 31 Principle of labeling syringe

Event-Based Learning Summary

The critical takeaway from this incident is the indispensable role of nurses in medication safety and patient care. While prompt responses and effective Code Blue activation are essential in emergencies, it is equally crucial to establish robust handover systems, adhere to strict medication labeling protocols, and foster a culture of seeking clarification when any doubt arises. Nurses must not administer any medications prepared by another nurse, unless it was prepared in their presence. Nurses should prioritize immediate patient assessment, than wasting time in checking monitor, tubings, ventilators etc.

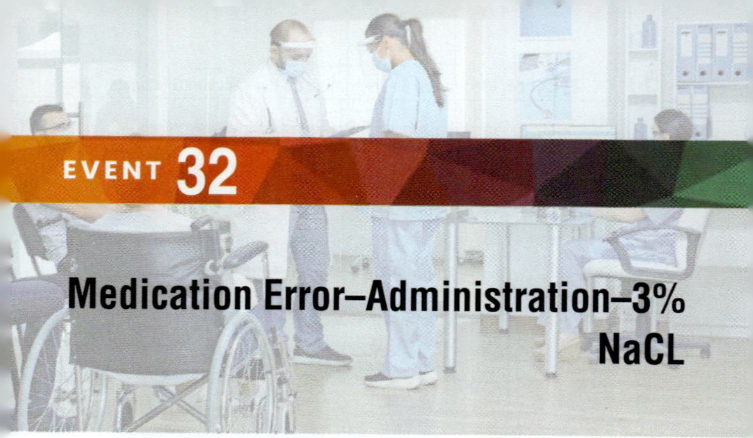

EVENT 32

Medication Error–Administration–3% NaCL

EVENT NO.	PSE/032/092022
IPSG RELATED TO	IPSG 3 – Safe Handling of High-Risk Medication

CASE STUDY DESCRIPTION

Mr Kishore, a 62-year-old patient, was admitted to the surgery ward, diagnosed with acute pancreatitis. The doctor prescribed Inj. Thiamine for the patient and, the assigned staff nurse administered Inj. Thiamine in 100 mL 3% NaCl instead of 100 mL 0.9% Normal Saline through the IV set. The senior nurse took round and observed the infusion and it was immediately stopped. Around 50 mL of infusion was administered by that time. She called the assigned nurse and showed the IV infusion. It was immediately informed to the duty consultant. Patient was observed and reassessed and the treatment plan was modified.

Positive Outcomes

- The senior nurse was alert and observed the infusion during the rounds.
- Immediately stopped the infusion as she was aware of the effect of 3% NaCl.

Errors Encountered

- The assigned nurse didn't follow the LASA drug policy.
- The nurse didn't check the saline strength before diluting.

- The nurse didn't follow rights of medications- proper preparation and administration.

Lessons Learned

For nurse	For nurse educator	For nurse administrator
• To have double verification for the medication administrations. • To remain diligent while using LASA medications and fluids. • Always ensure a second check by another nurse.	Train nurses on the list of LASA and high alert medications and orient them on the policy.	• Conduct periodic review and audit on LASA high alert medications and fluids. • Concentrated electrolytes including 3% NaCl are to be kept under lock. • Regular audit on storage, labeling and administration of high-alert medication

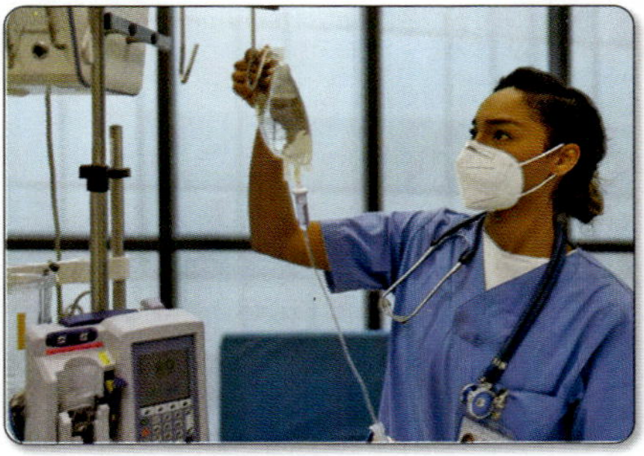

Figure 32 Double verification for medication administration

Event-Based Learning Summary

This medication error highlights the essential need for healthcare professionals to adhere to safety protocols, particularly the Look-alike Sound-alike (LASA) drug policy, to prevent errors related to medications with similar names. The vigilant senior nurse's actions in actively observing the infusion and promptly stopping the incorrect medication demonstrate the importance of vigilance. However, the assigned nurse's failure to follow proper medication verification, adherence to the rights of medication administration, and the LASA drug policy led to this error. The key lesson here is the paramount importance of rigorous adherence to established protocols and meticulous medication verification, preparation, and administration to ensure patient safety.

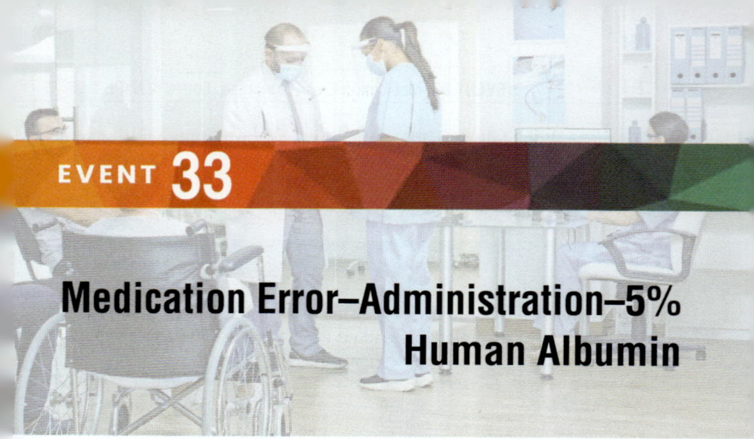

EVENT 33

Medication Error–Administration–5% Human Albumin

EVENT NO.	PSE/033/092022
IPSG RELATED TO	IPSG 3 – Safe Handling of High-Risk Medication

CASE STUDY DESCRIPTION

It was a typical busy day, and the morning duty nurse was asked to continue her duty as the scheduled second shift nurse did not report. She was assigned to look after a patient with Cirrhosis of liver. Inj. Human Albumin 250 mL (5%) was ordered, indented correctly, and delivered on time. The assigned nurse started Albumin infusion as soon as it reached. When the consultant came for rounds, he identified that instead of 250 mL, 500 mL of albumin was on flow.

Positive Outcome

Medicine administered on time without delay.

Errors Encountered

- All the 'rights' of medication administration were not followed.
- Right dose of drug not administered.
- Counter checking of high-alert medication was missed.

Lessons Learned

For nurse	For nurse educator	For nurse administrator
• To follow rights of medication administration. • To have double verification before administration of high-alert medication.	• To train and orient nurses on medication rights. • Emphasize safe practices of high-alert medications, especially two nurses verification.	• Audit medication administration practices periodically. • Regular audit on storage, labeling and administration of high-alert medication.

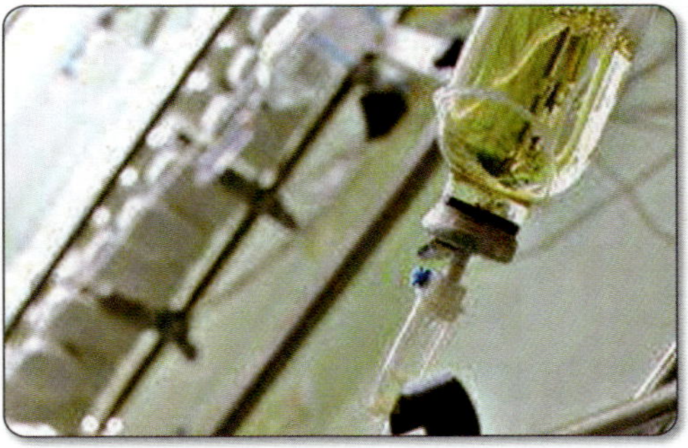

Figure 33 Albumin administration

Event-Based Learning Summary

In this medication error case, several important lessons emerge. While the nurse's volunteering attitude and timely medication administration are commendable, critical errors occurred. Not all the essential "rights" of medication administration were followed, resulting in the administration of the wrong medication dose—twice the prescribed amount. This incident underscores the utmost importance of adhering to established medication administration protocols, maintaining vigilance, and ensuring patient safety as the highest priority in healthcare. The need for two nurses verification for high-alert medications is paramount to prevent patient harm.

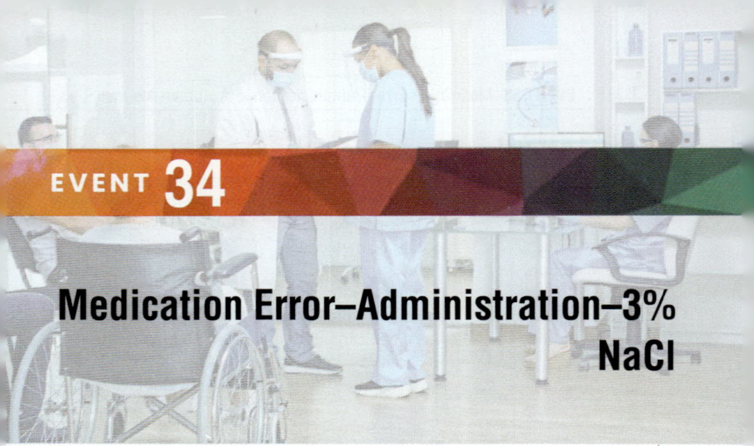

EVENT 34

Medication Error–Administration–3% NaCl

EVENT NO.	PSE/034/092022
IPSG RELATED TO	IPSG 3 – Safe Handling of High-Risk Medication

CASE STUDY DESCRIPTION

A 56-year-old patient, a known case of Diabetes Mellitus, on regular medications for the past 15 years, got admitted with complaints of swelling in legs, redness, and foot gangrene. The patient was found disoriented on the second day, and serum electrolytes revealed hyponatremia.

The report came in the evening, and the staff nurse on duty informed the values to the consultant over the phone. The doctor advised administering 3% Saline (hypertonic solution) 4 bottles over 24 hours. The concerned staff nurse handed over the patient to night duty staff and informed the orders but forgot to say the duration of infusion. The night staff administered the 3% Saline infusion, like normal IV fluids one by one over 12 hours and the solution finished within 12 hours. The error was identified during the morning handover, and immediately the intensivist was informed. The patient was closely monitored. After 2 hours, he developed ventricular tachycardia and collapsed. Immediately code blue paged, and the team successfully revived the patient.

Positive Outcomes

- The morning duty staff immediately identified and informed to the intensivist.
- The team was prepared to handle the situation as the complication was anticipated.

Errors Encountered

- Doctor ordered administration of high-risk medication over phone which was incomplete.
- The nurse failed to write down the telephonic order and read back for verification.
- The nurse also failed to get a complete order including duration/ infusion rate.
- Incoming nurse did not clarify the order.

Lessons Learned

For nurse	For nurse educator	For nurse administrator
• To follow rights of medication administration. • To have two-nurse verification before administration of high-alert medications. • To administer only against written orders except in Code Blue situation. • To be aware that IV fluids ordered over specific duration must be administered only after careful calculation of the drip rate.	• To train and orient nurses on medication rights. • Make them aware of medication errors related to high-alert medications and how to prevent them.	• Audit on medication administration periodically. • Regular audit on storage, labeling and administration of high-alert medication. • Privileging of nurses for medication administration must be adhered to.

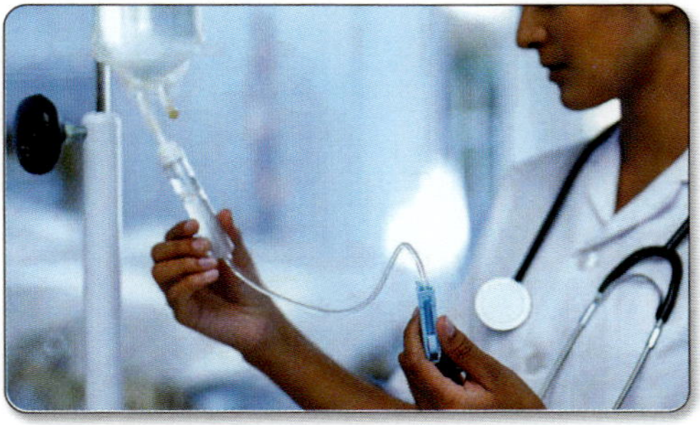

Figure 34 Nurse administering intravenous fluid in controlled rate

Event-Based Learning Summary

This medication error underscores critical lessons in healthcare. While the error was identified and managed, the incident reveals significant shortcomings. Nurses must be allowed to give medications, especially the high-alert medication only after privileging. Additionally, the practice of doctors providing medication orders via phone calls, especially for high-risk substances, without written documentation in the patient's file, is problematic. The nurse's failure to write down the telephonic order in patient's record and using Read-Back for verification further compounded the situation. This incident emphasizes the imperative of proper privileging of nurses for medication administration, close supervision, and the use of written orders to ensure patient safety in high-risk scenarios.

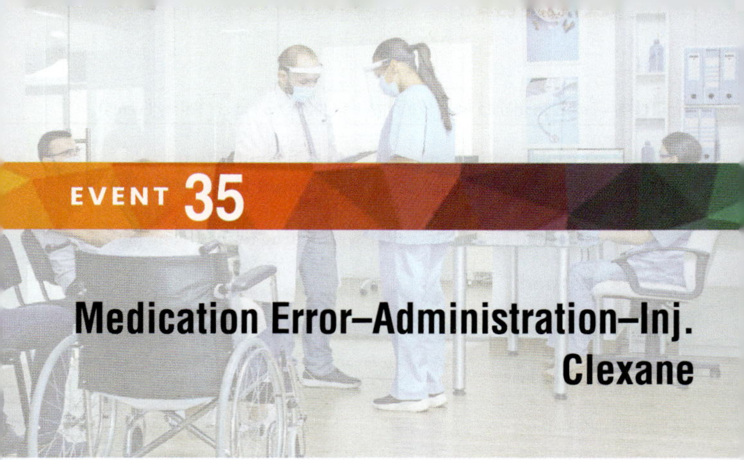

EVENT 35

Medication Error–Administration–Inj. Clexane

EVENT NO.	PSE/035/092022
IPSG RELATED TO	IPSG 3 – Safe Handling of High-Risk Medication

CASE STUDY DESCRIPTION

The senior nurse instructed the junior staff to administer the Inj. Clexane 60 mg to the patient, aged 65 years, diagnosed with DVT. The senior nurse told her the room number instead of the patient's name, and the junior staff took the medication without a medication chart and went to the room. Same time, another patient called her to disconnect the IV fluid. She went to the room and disconnected the IV fluid. When she came out of the room, she was confused about the room number. However, without checking with senior she entered the wrong room and administered Inj. Clexane 60 mg to a 45-year-old male patient who had undergone DJ stenting.

Positive Outcome

None.

Errors Encountered

- Verbal instruction was given for administering medication.
- The staff did not refer to the patient prescription before administering medication.
- Did not identify the patient by using two identifiers along with the medication chart.

- There were interruptions during medication administration.
- Staff never bothered to recheck with the team leader when she had confusion.
- She assumed and administered the wrong drug to the wrong patient.

Lessons Learned

For nurse	For nurse educator	For nurse administrator
• To follow rights of medication administration. • To have two nurses verification before administration of high alert medications. • Never to use room numbers as identifiers. • Verbal instructions from another nurse should never be followed. • Always ensure that nurse should carry medication chart to the bedside to identify the patient correctly before administering medication.	• To train and orient nurses on medication rights. • Train them using simulation scenarios to emphasize potential harm when safe practices are not followed.	• Audit on medication administration periodically. • Any deviation in the process should be encouraged to be reported. • When doing RCA of such events always ensure the front line nurses involved in the event are invited to participate.

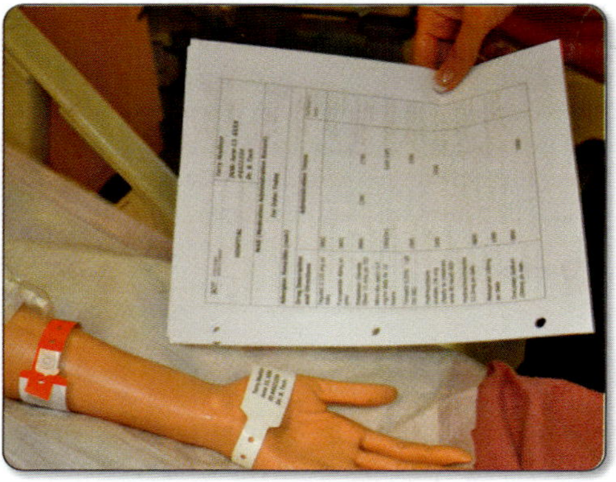

Figure 35 Safe medication administration after cross checking with UHID number

Event-Based Learning Summary

While errors occurred at various stages, the most crucial takeaway is the unwavering need to follow standard medication administration protocols. Verbal instructions for medication should never be taken from another nurse and checking the patient's prescription is paramount. Proper patient identification, using at least two identifiers, and minimizing interruptions during medication administration are essential safeguards. Equally important is the culture of self-checking and seeking clarification when any doubt arises. This incident emphasizes that at no stage of medication administration should our guard be lowered, and unwavering adherence to established protocols remains the cornerstone of patient safety.

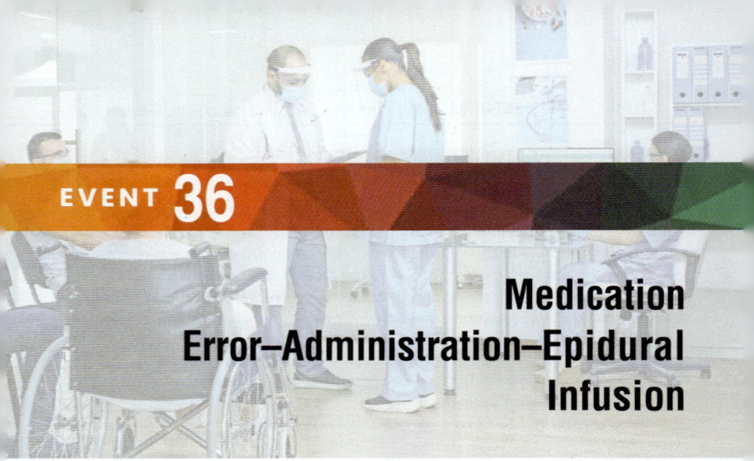

EVENT 36

Medication Error–Administration–Epidural Infusion

EVENT NO.	PSE/036/092022
IPSG RELATED TO	IPSG 3 – Safe Handling of High-Risk Medication

CASE STUDY DESCRIPTION

A 64-year-old female patient who had undergone a right total knee replacement was shifted to the ward with an epidural infusion. During the clinical rounds, the patient complained of pain to the in-charge nurse and asked for pain medication. The in-charge nurse instructed the concerned staff about the patient complaint and asked her to connect the epidural infusion as she was unaware of the flow rate. Instead of going to the patient's room and connecting the line, the concerned nurse asked another junior nurse to do the same. The junior nurse connected the infusion to the IV line instead of the epidural line.

Positive Outcome

None.

Errors Encountered

- There were multiple passes of verbal information between the staff without documenting.
- In-charge failed to cross-check the flow rate from the concerned nurse or the case sheet.

- Senior staff instructed the assigned nurse to go and connect the line (never instructed about the epidural line) as she was attending another doctor's rounds.
- Failed to cross-check with the staff if she is aware of the epidural line connection.
- The assigned nurse assumed that the epidural is to be connected to the IV line as it was through an infusion pump.
- Junior staff failed to read the caution sticker on the line, which clearly stated "Epidural Line".
- The concerned nurse never thought to cross-check whether the assigned nurse has connected to the correct route.

Lessons Learned

For nurse	For nurse educator	For nurse administrator
• Verbal instruction on medication administration must NOT be followed. • Always administer medication after verifying doctor's prescription at the bedside to ensure all Rights of medications are complied with.	• To train and orient nurses on medication rights. • Make them aware on medication errors and SOPs to prevent them. • Special training and privileging should be done on epidural infusion.	• Implement safe SOP for handing epidural lines. • To ensure the availability of color-coded label and caution stickers in the department. • Audit on epidural medication administration periodically.

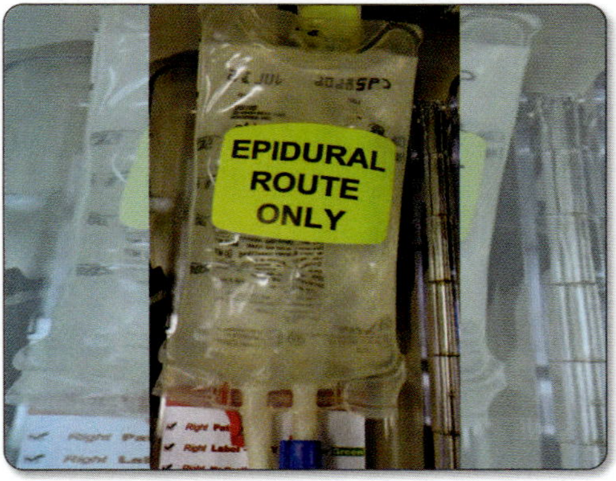

Figure 36 Epidural infusion should be marked

Event-Based Learning Summary

This medication error incident highlights crucial lessons in medication administration process. A primary takeaway is the absolute importance of not accepting verbal medication orders, especially from senior nurses, without clear and documented instructions. Relying solely on verbal communication can lead to misunderstandings and errors. In this case, the failure to cross-check the medication route and a lack of diligence in reading warning labels resulted in a critical error. Nurses should always prioritize written and well-documented orders to ensure medication administration accuracy, emphasizing the significance of double-checking procedures to maintain patient safety.

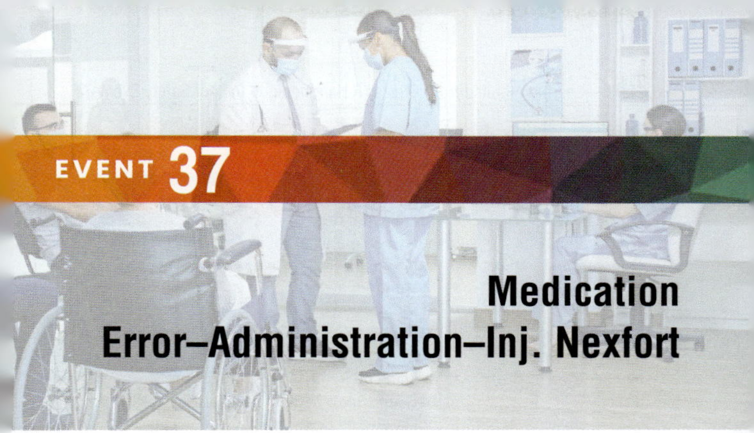

EVENT 37

Medication Error–Administration–Inj. Nexfort

EVENT NO.	PSE/037/092022
IPSG RELATED TO	None

CASE STUDY DESCRIPTION

The doctor ordered Inj. Cedocef TZ 2.25 g, a nonformulary medicine, which was unavailable in the pharmacy. Team leader confirmed with the doctor, which was advised giving Inj. Nexfort TZ 2.5 g BD over the phone. Medication was transcribed as Inj. Nexfort 2.25 g (wrong transcription), Indented TZ 1.5 g (wrong indent), and two wrong doses were administered (wrong administration).

Positive Outcome

Disastrous results of wrong medication did not happen.

Errors Encountered

- Nurses did not follow the rights of medication administration.
- Team leader took the verbal order and shared it with the duty doctor resulting in wrong transcription and indent.
- Telephonic order protocol Read-Back and Spell-Back was not followed.

Lessons Learned

For nurse	For nurse educator	For nurse administrator
• Verbal orders are taken only in emergency situations (Code Blue). • Telephonic medication orders better be taken by doctor on duty directly. • In case of unavoidable situations, the nurse must right the order in the patient's file and Read-Back/Spell-Back to ensure they have received the correct orders.	• To train and orient nurses on medication rights. • Make them aware of medication errors and SOPs to prevent them. • Training on Read-Back and Spell-Back policy should be taught through simulation-based scenarios.	• Ensure the policy on verbal and telephonic orders are clearly understood by all concerned. • Audit on telephonic orders and Read-Back procedure must be conducted periodically.

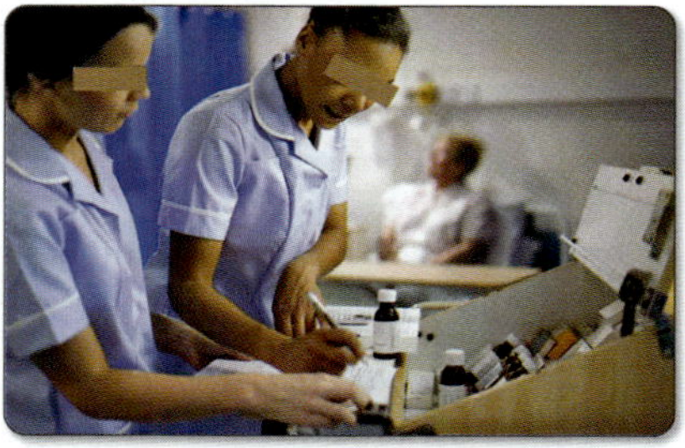

Figure 37 Wrong medication transcribed by nurse

Event-Based Learning Summary

In this medication error scenario, the failure to follow the established process of telephonic orders led to significant issues. Nurses did not adhere to the proper procedures, resulting in the wrong transcription and indent of the medication. Furthermore, the neglect of the telephonic order protocol exacerbated the situation. While the patient was fortunate to escape disastrous consequences, this incident underscores the critical importance of strict adherence to medication administration protocols, clear communication, and proper procedures in healthcare practice to ensure patient safety.

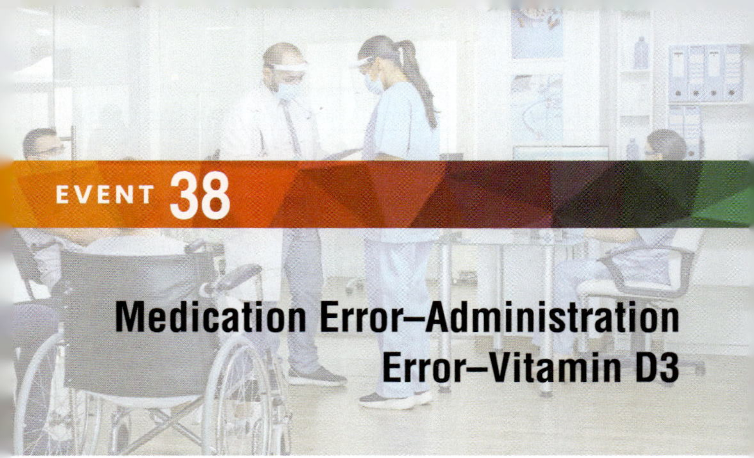

EVENT 38

Medication Error–Administration Error–Vitamin D3

EVENT NO.	PSE/038/092022
IPSG RELATED TO	None

CASE STUDY DESCRIPTION

The doctor prescribed Capsule Vitamin D3 PO 60,000 IU per week for 6 weeks. The nurse wrote the schedule as 6th hourly in the medication chart and administered one extra dose the next day.

Positive Outcome

The patient got only one additional dose.

Errors Encountered

- The drug frequency for 6 weeks was perceived as 6th hourly by the nurse.
- The nurse did not reconfirm with the concerned doctor or TL.
- The nurse transcribed the wrong frequency of the medication, resulting in one extra dose in the patient.

Lessons Learned

For nurse	For nurse educator	For nurse administrator
• It is always prudent to check the doctor's order as well when the medication is transcribed by the nurses. • Make an effort to know the drugs which nurse is administering (action, dose, route, frequency and side-effects).	• To train and orient nurses on medication rights. • Make them aware of medication errors and SOPs to prevent them.	• Ensure the policy is requiring doctor to write the medication orders directly in the medication chart. • To institute a policy which prohibits the nurses from transcribing the doctor's order.

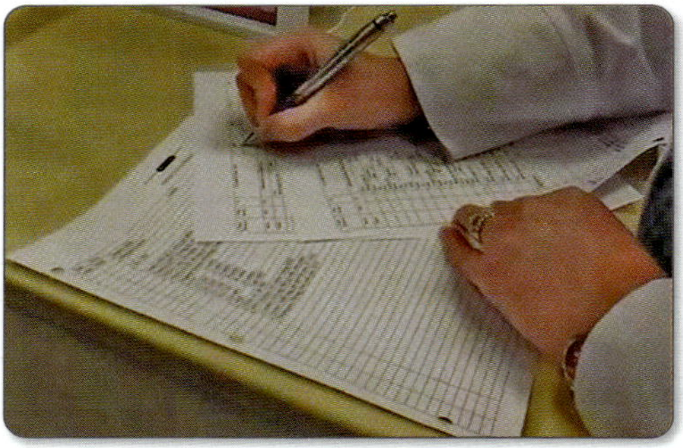

Figure 38 Doctor prescribing the medication in the medication chart

Event-Based Learning Summary

This event highlights a crucial lesson that nurses must possess a comprehensive understanding of typical medication doses. When in doubt, it is imperative to seek clarification from the prescribing doctor and consult the drug formulary. In this case, a misinterpretation of the dosage frequency occurred, leading to an erroneous dosing schedule and the administration of an extra dose. To prevent such errors, healthcare professionals should always ensure they are well-informed about medication dosages, and when unsure, seek guidance to guarantee accurate medication administration. The medication administration policy must insist on doctor's writing the medication order directly into the medication chart, thereby avoiding transcription errors.

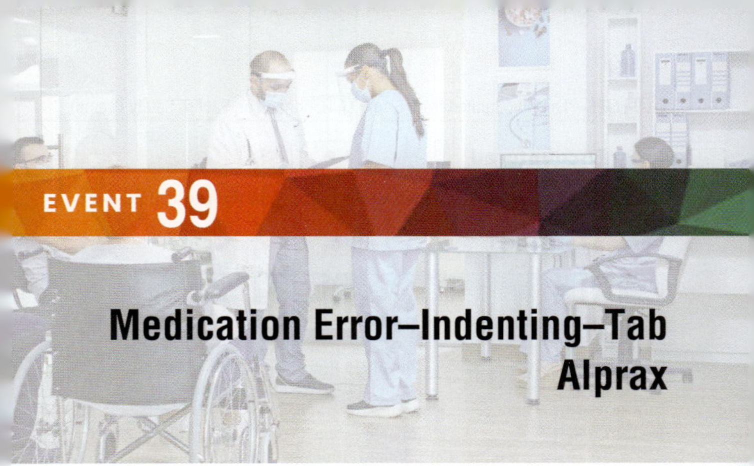

EVENT 39

Medication Error–Indenting–Tab Alprax

EVENT NO.	PSE/039/092022
IPSG RELATED TO	IPSG 3 – Safe Handling of High-Risk Medication

CASE STUDY DESCRIPTION

A 25-year-old woman came to the hospital complaining of joint pain and intermittent lower back pain. Also, she informed the nurse that she has trouble falling asleep at night and cannot get a good night's rest. She has been constantly worried about her performance at her workplace, with her family, and toward her mother's health. She feels tensed most of the day, causing her to feel stiff. She also has difficulty paying attention to her work and finishing her assigned job. After hearing the complains, the doctor prescribed Tab Alprax (0.5 mg) and told her to follow-up after one week. The nurse entered the medicines into the system for indenting from the pharmacy. She entered Tab. Alprax 5 mg instead of 0.5 mg. The next day patient came with the complains of severe drowsiness, confusion, and slurred speech. Upon further inquiry it was found that the patient had taken Tab. Alprax 5 mg instead of 0.5 mg.

Positive Outcome

None.

Error Encountered

The patient ended up taking ten times more than the prescribed dose.

Lessons Learned

For nurse	For nurse educator	For nurse administrator
• Have knowledge on the drugs that are being intended. • Verify with seniors or doctors in case of any doubt.	• To train and orient nurses on medication that are in the formulary. • Ensure the training on medication administration focuses on High-Alert mediations available in the hospital.	• To work with the IT department to flag any medication indent which are outside the permissible limits. • Ensure nurses are privileged for medication administration specifically for high-alert medications.

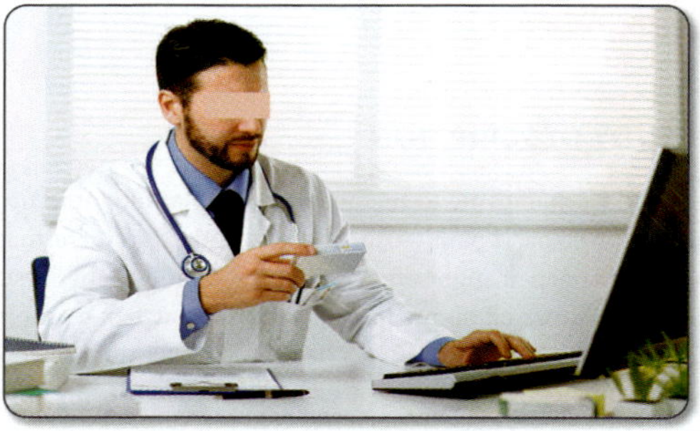

Figure 39 Doctor prescribing and indenting the medication, avoiding medication errors

Event-Based Learning Summary

In this case, a nurse's misunderstanding of the prescribed dosage resulted in the patient receiving 10 times the intended medication, leading to severe drowsiness and confusion. This also emphasized the need for nurses to be aware of the usual doses of medications. This will prompt them to question an erroneous order. To enhance patient safety, healthcare professionals must exercise meticulous attention to detail, ensuring that the right medications are prescribed and administered accurately.

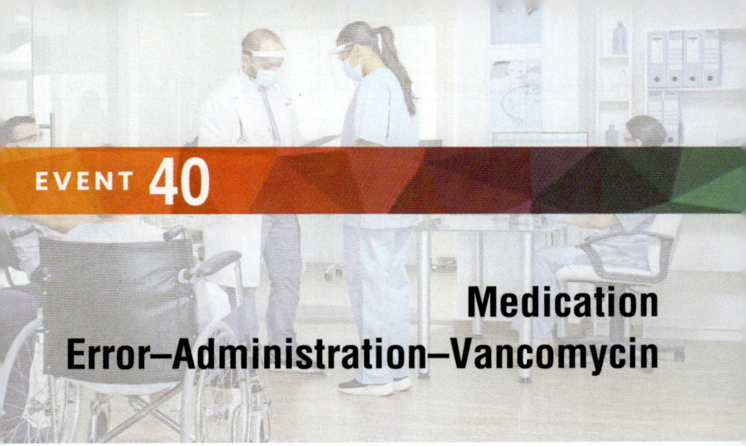

EVENT 40

Medication Error–Administration–Vancomycin

EVENT NO.	PSE/040/092022
IPSG RELATED TO	IPSG 3 – Safe Handling of High-Risk Medication

CASE STUDY DESCRIPTION

A 61-year-old patient was admitted to the hospital in the haemato-oncology ward. He was prescribed Inj. Vancomycin 1 g intravenous (IV) BD without mentioning the dilution. The standard dilution recommended is Inj Vancomycin in 200 mL normal saline. But the patient received 1 g Vancomycin in 100 mL normal saline making the concentration 10 mg/mL which is higher than the recommended dilution.

Positive Outcome

The error did not result in any adverse effects on the patient.

Errors Encountered

- Incomplete order from the doctor.
- Incorrect drug dilution.
- Wrong rate of administration.

Lessons Learned

For nurse	For nurse educator	For nurse administrator
• Nurses must insist on a complete prescription with drug name, dose, route, frequency, and dilution. • While documenting, write down the actual amount of dilution with medication. • Be mindful during the dilution of medication. • Recheck the calculation to ensure that the patient gets the correct therapeutic dose. • Double-check the dosing and frequency of high-alert medications. • Get one more nurse to check the high-alert medications before administration.	• To train and orient nurses on medication that are in the formulary. • Ensure the training on medication administration focuses on High-Alert mediations available in the hospital.	• Printed dilution table to be made available as ready reckoner in all nurse's stations. • Privileging of nurses for medication administration must be adhered to.

VANCOMYCIN DOSING AND INFUSION TIME [note maximum rate of infusion = 10 mg/min (600 mg/hr)]			
Patient's Weight	**Dose**	**Infusion time and volume**	**Ideally commence infusion**
42–58 kg	750 mg	75 minutes in 250 mL NS	85–105 minutes prior to skin incision
59–74 kg	1000 mg	100 minutes in 250 mL NS	110–130 minutes prior to skin incision
75–91 kg	1250 mg	125 minutes in 250 mL NS	135–155 minutes prior to skin incision
92–108 kg	1500 mg	150 minutes in 250 mL NS	160–180 minutes prior to skin incision
109–124 kg	1750 mg	175 minutes in 500 mL NS	185–205 minutes prior to skin incision
≥125 kg	2000 mg	200 minutes in 500 mL NS	210–230 minutes prior to skin incision

Figure 40 Inj. Vancomycin dosing and infusion time

Event-Based Learning Summary

This medication error underscores the vital importance of nurses having a comprehensive understanding of medications and their dilution protocols. When facing unfamiliar medications or uncertainties, it is paramount to seek guidance from a senior or a knowledgeable colleague. Medication errors can have irreversible consequences, potentially causing serious harm to patients. Therefore, nurses must prioritize their ongoing education, continuously enhancing their knowledge and skills. When in doubt, asking questions and seeking clarification is not only encouraged but essential for ensuring patient safety.

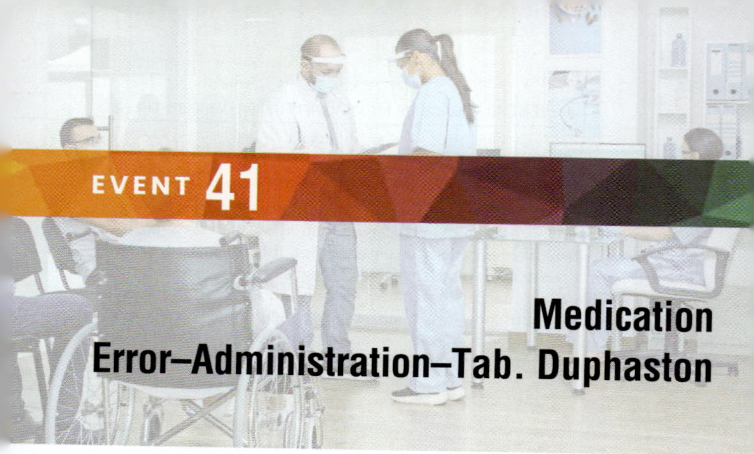

EVENT 41

Medication Error–Administration–Tab. Duphaston

EVENT NO.	PSE/041/092022
IPSG RELATED TO	None

CASE STUDY DESCRIPTION

A 34-year-old patient got admitted for antenatal care as she is a high-risk mother. The mother developed hypertension during pregnancy and was diagnosed as elderly primi with PIH. The doctor prescribed Tab. Duphaston 20 mg OD. But while administering medication, the nurse gave only 10 mg because the available form of Tab. Duphaston in the pharmacy was 10 mg/tablet. The patient has been taking this medication since the second trimester, so she knows she must take two tablets. The patient attender came to the nurses' station and inquired about the dosage of the tablet. Only then the nurse realized that she has to give two tablets for 20 mg. Then the nurse immediately gave the second tablet to the patient.

Positive Outcomes

- The patient attender reported to the nurses' station as they knew the correct dosage of the tablet since they had been taking it for a long time.
- Alert and timely reporting by the attender, prevented any adverse event due to suboptimal dose of Tab. Duphaston.

- The nurse accepted the error and ensured timely correction by administering the correct dose of medication.

Errors Encountered

- The nurse did not check for the right dosage in the order.
- The nurse did not explain the medications and their dosage.
- An alert from the pharmacy on the non-availability of the prescribed strength was not done.

Lessons Learned

For nurse	For nurse educator	For nurse administrator
• The nurse should check the dosage in the doctor's order and the available form of the medicine (name, strength, dose, and route). • Involving patient in the medication administration by explaining the action and dose of medicines can prevent such errors.	• All nurses to be trained on the process of double verification. • Train nurses to involve patient and family members in their care. "Nothing about me, without me".	• The SOP on double verification process to be created/ strengthened. • Periodic audits on safe medication management to be conducted.

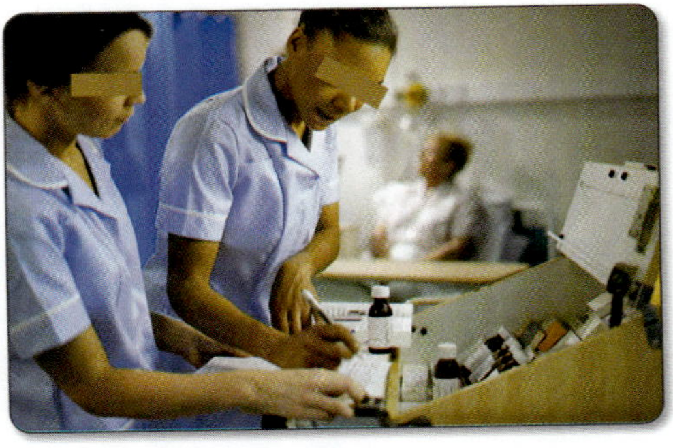

Figure 41 Nurses check and verify the medication (name, strength, dose and route)

Event-Based Learning Summary

In this case, the patient's active involvement in her care and the timely reporting by her attendant prevented a potentially life-threatening situation. The patient knew the correct dosage due to her prior experience with the medication, which highlights the importance of patient education. However, the nurse failed to verify the prescribed dosage, emphasizing the need for healthcare providers to double-check medication orders for accuracy. Moreover, the absence of an alert from the pharmacy regarding the unavailability of the prescribed strength contributed to this error, highlighting the significance of effective communication in healthcare settings. Mistakes can happen, but it is crucial for nurses to acknowledge and rectify them promptly, ensuring patient safety remains the top priority.

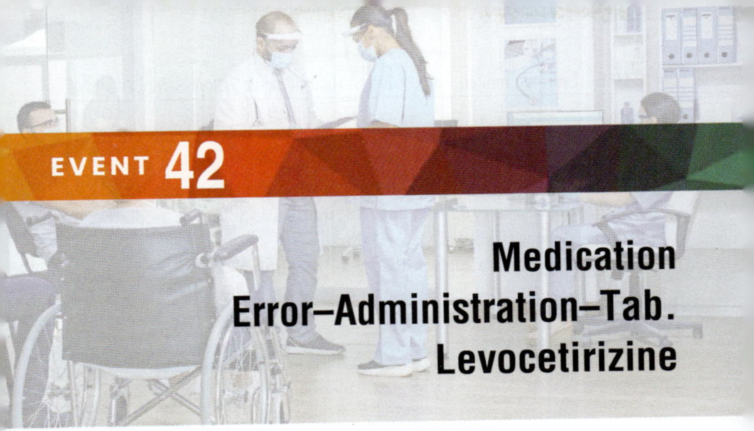

EVENT 42

Medication Error–Administration–Tab. Levocetirizine

EVENT NO.	PSE/042/092022
IPSG RELATED TO	None

CASE STUDY DESCRIPTION

A 9-year-old child with a known case of acute Lymphoblastic Leukemia was admitted for scheduled chemotherapy with Inj. Vincristine. The child was also given another supportive medication as per the doctor's prescription, Tab. Levocetirizine 1 tab 0-0-1, as mentioned in the treatment chart. The nursing staff administered Tab. Levocetirizine 1 tablet of 10 mg, but the recommended dose for children between 6 and 11 years is 2.5 mg once a day.

Positive Outcomes

- The child did not develop any symptoms of overdosage of Tab. Levocetirizine.
- Error was caught on time and patient was monitored until discharge.

Errors Encountered

- An incomplete and incorrect prescription of the dose of the medication.
- Elements of prescription not followed.

- Not involving a clinical pharmacist who can double-check the prescription.
- Indenting the medication without knowing the right strength.
- Dispensing the wrong strength of medication to the pediatric age group. There was no drug oversight.
- The child received a higher dose than recommended.

Lessons Learned

For nurse	For nurse educator	For nurse administrator
Never carry out incomplete prescriptions, insist on a complete and accurate prescription with name of drug, route, dose and frequency.	• Staffs to be trained on pediatric drug dose preparations/age specific doses. • Training nurses not to carry out orders written as just tablets and ampoules. They must ask for a complete prescription—name, strength, dose, and route.	• Age-specific competency training must be implemented before posting nurses to pediatric department. • Privileging nurses for the medication administration. • Clear escalation matrix for an incomplete prescription.

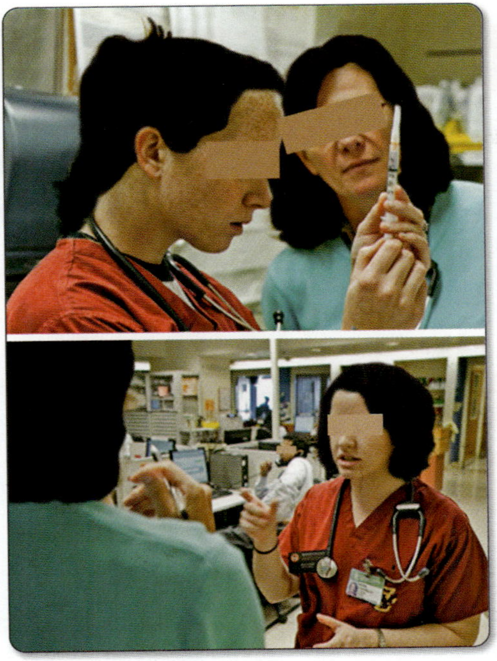

Figure 42 Double checking the medication at all levels

Event-Based Learning Summary

In this case, multiple errors occurred in the prescription and administration of medication to a 9-year-old child undergoing chemotherapy. The prescribed dose of Tab. Levocetirizine was incorrect and exceeded the appropriate dosage for the child's age group, illustrating the importance of precise prescription details and adhering to established pediatric dosing guidelines. On the positive side, the child did not experience any symptoms of medication overdose, and healthcare providers promptly recognized the error, initiating vigilant monitoring until discharge. To prevent such errors, healthcare teams should prioritize complete and accurate prescriptions and involve clinical pharmacists for double-checking medication orders, ensuring the safety of pediatric patients.

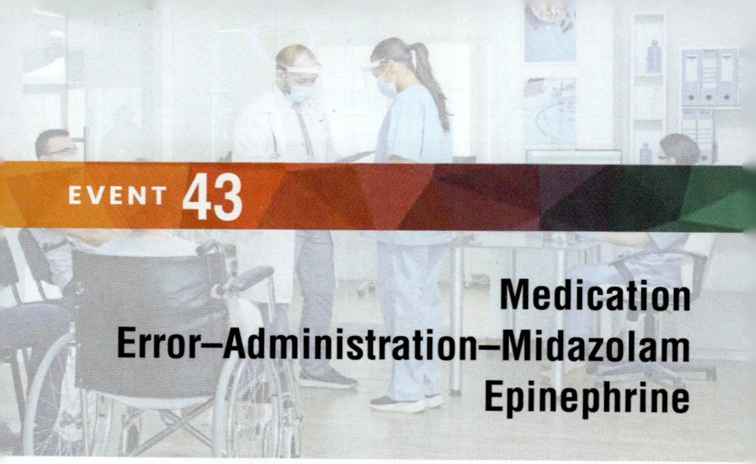

EVENT 43

Medication Error–Administration–Midazolam Epinephrine

EVENT NO.	PSE/043/092022
IPSG RELATED TO	IPSG 3 – Safe Handling of High-Risk Medication

CASE STUDY DESCRIPTION

A 50-year-old woman presented to the hospital with a history of abdominal pain and altered bowel habits. A colonoscopy was scheduled for the following day. Before the colonoscopy, the doctor advised the assisting nurse to administer Inj. Midazolam 5 mg. In a hurry, the nurse took an ampoule of Inj. Epinephrine and administered the same. After receiving Inj. Epinephrine, the patient complained of chest tightness, difficulty breathing, and generalized tremors. The doctor postponed the procedure and asked the nurse what dose of Inj. Midazolam she had administered. During the inventory check, it was discovered that the attending nurse administered 0.25 mg of Epinephrine instead of Inj. Midazolam. The ampoules were kept together, and the nurse missed to cross-check the medication before administering it to the patient. The procedure was postponed for several days until the patient recovered.

Positive Outcome

The patient could be saved by timely recognition of the medication error.

Errors Encountered

- The high-alert medications were kept together.
- The nurse did not cross-check the Inj. before taking it out of the cart, before withdrawing, and before administration.
- While checking the cart, the nurse missed noticing that these medications were kept together.

Lessons Learned

For nurse	For nurse educator	For nurse administrator
• Always follow written orders only. • Two nurses must verify all high-alert medications administration. • When checking cart, identify risky area (in this case Medaz & Epi being kept side by side) and escalate to the seniors to remedy the concerns.	• Rigorous training at all levels (physicians, nurses, pharmacists) on safely handling high alert medications. • All healthcare workers, especially nurses, must be trained on human factors to sensitize them that while handling high-alert medication, a double check by one more person is mandatory and is a safe practice.	• Define policy on prescription, dispensing, administration, and storage of high alert medications. • High alert medication of various classes and strengths cannot be kept "together" as described in the event. • Quality improvement projects need to be implemented to avoid such errors in the future after a proper RCA.

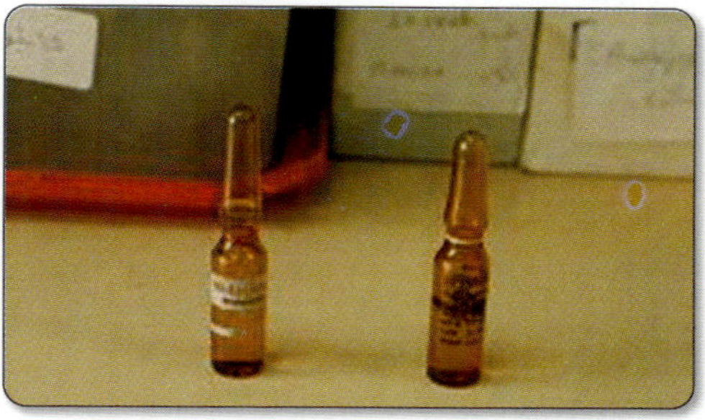

Figure 43 Epinephrine ampoule and Midazolam ampoule

Event-Based Learning Summary

In this case, a serious medication error occurred when a nurse mistakenly administered Inj. Epinephrine instead of the prescribed Inj. Midazolam to a patient scheduled for a colonoscopy. The medications were stored together contributing to the error, highlighting the importance of appropriate medication storage and organization. The nurse failed to cross-check the medication before withdrawal and administration, underscoring the critical role of verification in preventing such errors. Fortunately, the patient was saved due to the timely recognition of the mistake, and the procedure was postponed until the patient fully recovered. Healthcare providers should prioritize safe medication practices, including proper medication storage and vigilant double-checking procedures to ensure patient safety.

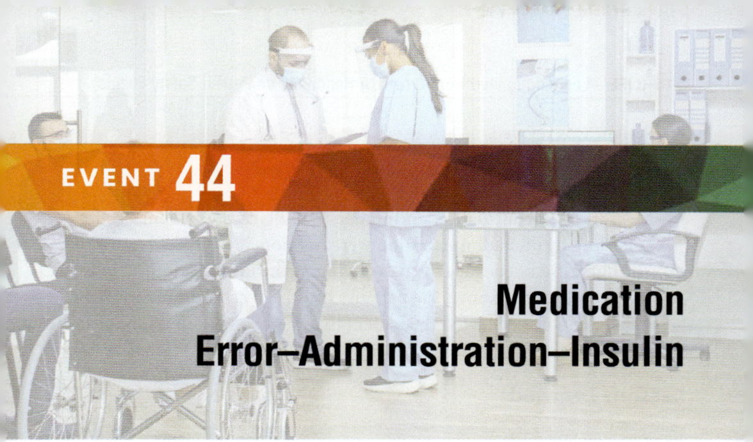

EVENT 44

Medication Error–Administration–Insulin

EVENT NO.	PSE/044/092022
IPSG RELATED TO	IPSG 3 – Safe Handling of High-Risk Medication

CASE STUDY DESCRIPTION

A 50-year-old female patient had diabetes for 20 years. She has been on regular oral hypoglycemic agents (OHAs). Since the blood sugar was uncontrolled with the OHAs, she was prescribed Inj. Huminsulin (R) thrice a day (10 U – 12 U – 7 U). She was taught to self-administer Inj. Insulin. Even after this, the blood sugar were uncontrolled, so she was admitted to a medical center. On the first day of admission, the patient took 10 U with breakfast at 7:30 am.

At 7:45 am, the assigned nurse measured the patient's blood sugar, which was 289 mg/dL; and the value was informed to the patient. At 7:50 am, the same nurse administered Inj. Huminsulin (R) 10 U. The patient obliged and did not notify the nurse of taking the regular dose at 7:30 am since she assumed it was a part of the hospital treatment. At 8:15 am, after her breakfast, the patient became restless; she started sweating profusely, her skin became cold and clammy, and finally, she became unresponsive. Her blood sugar dropped to 32 mg/dL. The same nurse intervened promptly, with intravenous Dextrose and the patient was revived.

Positive Outcomes

- Nurse acted promptly.

- Patient was revived.

Errors Encountered

- Medication reconciliation and understanding of the patient's routine regarding insulin administration were not done.
- The nurse did not engage the patient during the insulin administration.
- The nurse neither knows the patient's history of self-administration of Insulin and nor educated the patient that in hospital, nurses should be administering all medications.

Lessons Learned

For nurse	For nurse educator	For nurse administrator
• Patient must be educated on medication administration timing and policy. • Patient and patient's family members must be educated at the time of admission to refrain from any self-administration of medication in the hospital.	• Train nurse on medication policies including self-administration of medication. • Discuss the scenario during training and highlight to educate patients/attendants on the policy of self-medication at hospital.	• To have home medication reconciliation and self-medication administration policy. • Medications are to be kept under lock and key.

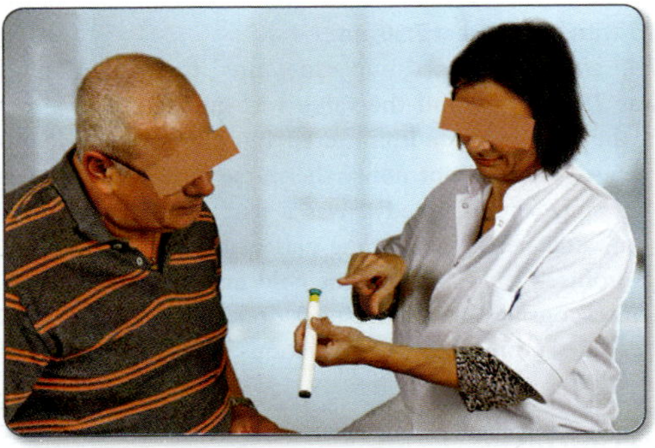

Figure 44 Nurse explaining how to use insulin pen

Event-Based Learning Summary

In this case, a medication error occurred due to a lack of proper medication reconciliation and communication with the patient. A 50-year-old diabetic patient, who had been self-administering Inj. Huminsulin (R) at home, experienced a life-threatening situation. The nurse assigned to the patient failed to engage in a conversation with the patient regarding her insulin routine and did not explain the hospital's medication administration procedures. This lack of communication led to the patient receiving an additional dose of insulin causing her blood sugar levels to drop significantly. Fortunately, the nurse acted promptly to revive the patient. This case underscores the critical importance of medication reconciliation and effective patient communication to ensure safe and accurate medication administration, particularly for patients with pre-existing medication regimens.

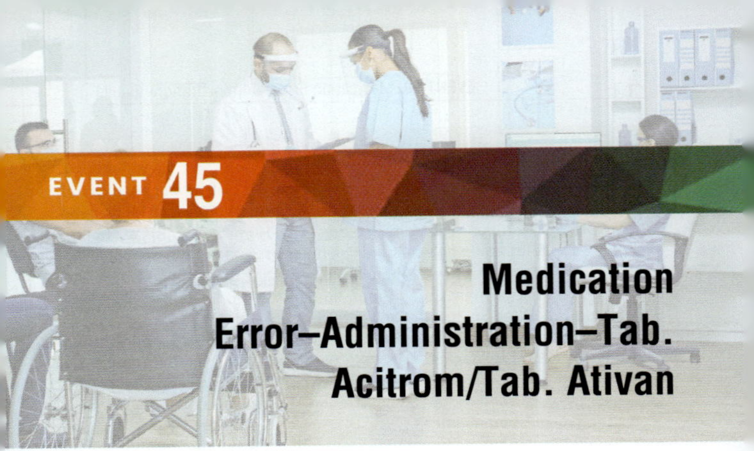

EVENT 45

Medication Error–Administration–Tab. Acitrom/Tab. Ativan

EVENT NO.	PSE/045/092022
IPSG RELATED TO	IPSG 3 – Safe Handling of High-Risk Medication

CASE STUDY DESCRIPTION

Mr Kumaresan, a 56-year-old male patient admitted in male medical ward, diagnosed with DVT. The treating doctor prescribed Tab. Acitrom 1 mg as morning dose. The assigned nurse transcribed the medicine and asked the patient attendant to buy the drug from the pharmacy and come back. After receiving the drug, the staff nurse administered the medicine. After 40 minutes, the patient complained of itching all over the body. The nurse immediately informed the treating doctor and reassessment was done. The team found that the patient had developed an allergic drug reaction because the nurse had administered Tab. Ativan instead of Tab. Acitrom. Tab. Ativan caused allergy to that patient.

Positive Outcome

The assigned nurse immediately escalated the incident to the treating consultant.

Errors Encountered

- The nurse transcribed the wrong medicine.
- The nurse failed to verify the medicine with the prescription.

Lessons Learned

For nurse	For nurse educator	For nurse administrator
• Have knowledge on the drugs that are being administered. • Verify with seniors or doctors in case of doubt. • Follow rights of medication administration.	• To train and orient nurses on medication that are in the formulary. • Make them aware on medication errors and SOPs to prevent them.	• To have a process of indenting from the prescription directly instead of entering it again by a second person from prescription. • Ensure that all high-alert medications are checked by two nurses before administration, after verifying the order for the right patient.

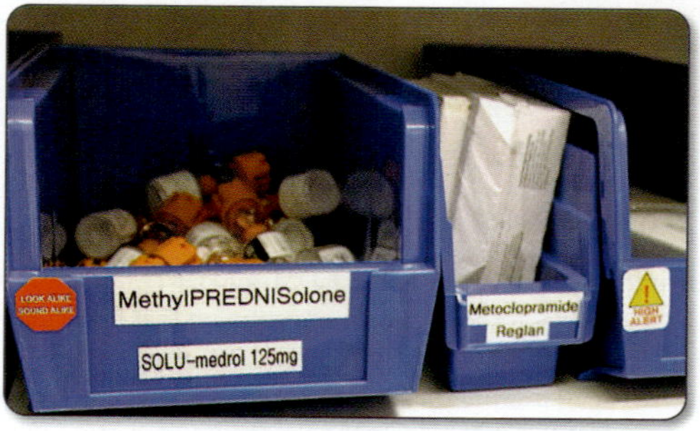

Figure 45 Storage of LASA drugs separately to prevent medication error

Event-Based Learning Summary

In this case, a medication error occurred when a 56-year-old male patient was diagnosed with DVT and prescribed Tab. Acitrom 1 mg. The nurse mistakenly administered Tab. Ativan to the patient resulting in an allergic drug reaction. The error was promptly recognized when the patient complained of itching, and the nurse escalated the incident to the treating consultant. Immediate re-assessment was conducted, preventing further complications. However, this case highlights the importance of adhering to the LASA drug administration protocol and the rights of medication to avoid such errors and ensure patient safety. Additionally, nurses should maintain a strong knowledge of medications and their specific indications for each patient while always double-checking their actions to prevent medication errors.

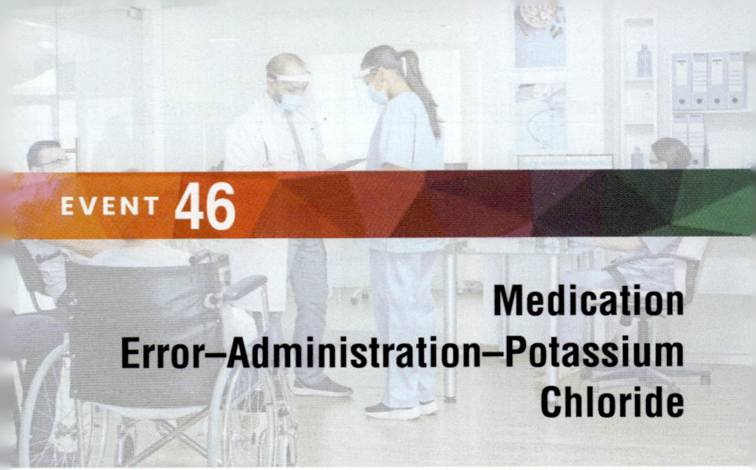

EVENT 46

Medication Error–Administration–Potassium Chloride

EVENT NO.	PSE/046/092022
IPSG RELATED TO	IPSG 3 – Safe Handling of High-Risk Medication

CASE STUDY DESCRIPTION

A 62-year-old male patient with CAD, DM, and CKD was admitted to the medical ICU. He was for Potassium correction on that particular day. The doctor ordered Inj. Potassium Chloride IV infusion, 40 mEq in 40 mL dilution (NS) at 10 mL/hr. The patient was assigned to a pull-in staff. The duty doctor asked the staff to start the Potassium correction immediately with 40 mEq Potassium Chloride. The nurse loaded 2 ampoules (20 mEq each) of Potassium Chloride and injected *via* arterial line. While administering the patient was screaming with pain and irritation in his hand. The duty doctor attended patient immediately and recognized the patient had received Inj. Potassium Chloride *via* arterial line. The infusion was stopped immediately. The incident was investigated and found that the assigned nurse had no prior critical care experience and never handled any invasive lines. The in-charge nurse of ICU had not checked with the pull-in nurse about her critical care/clinical experience before assigning her to a patient with multiple lines.

Positive Outcome

None.

Errors Encountered

- Undiluted potassium chloride was administered *via* arterial line.
- Written doctor's order was not reviewed by the assigned nurse.
- Two-nurse verification was not done for the high-alert medication (Potassium Chloride)
- Senior nurses failed to verify the experience and competency of pull-in staff.
- Adequate supervision was not provided to the pull-in staff.
- The lines were not labeled to provide caution alert.

Lessons Learned

For nurse	For nurse educator	For nurse administrator
• Ask for help when a nurse is assigned to unfamiliar nursing care department. • Be assertive and verbalize if encountered with procedures the nurse has never done before. • Adhere to the policy on the handling of concentrated electrolytes. • When taking over patients, check all lines for correct position and label.	• Ask for help when in doubt must be emphasized during the training to the nurses to prevent unintended harm of patient. • Such incidents can be discussed during training to sensitize nurses about the potential harm they can cause when they are pulled out for unfamiliar nursing departments.	• Have a policy emphasizing that the nurses with no experience in critical care must not be on pulled out. • Experienced nurses when pulled-out in the other critical care departments, mini orientation to the unit and supervision must be provided. • Job delegation must be based on the competency level required for the particular department. • Audit pull-in, pull-out process to ensure right skilled nurse to the right patient.

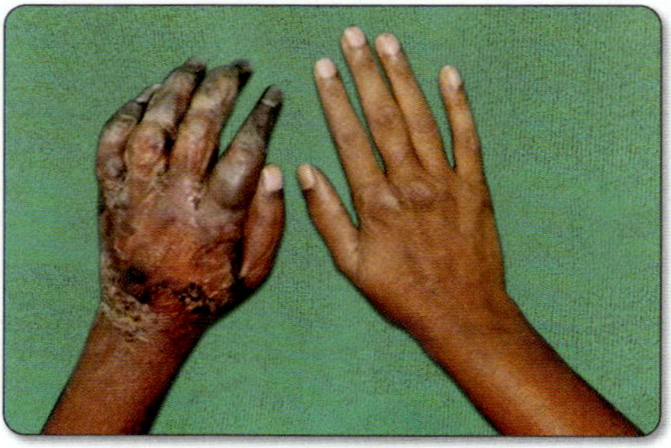

Figure 46 Consequence of administering intravenous medication to the radial arterial line

Event-Based Learning Summary

In this case, a 62-year-old male patient with a history of CAD, DM and CKD was admitted to a medical ICU for treatment, which included potassium correction. Unfortunately, a series of errors occurred during the administration of Inj. Potassium Chloride resulting in patient harm. The assignment of a new nurse without critical care experience from another department to the ICU was the initial misstep. This nurse was not adequately assessed or supervised, highlighting a lack of proper job delegation and induction processes. The nurse mistakenly administered concentrated Inj. Potassium 40 mEq into the arterial line, causing severe pain and distress to the patient. Notably, no double-check was performed before administration, and the lines were not appropriately labeled. This case underscores the critical importance of proper staffing, training, supervision, and double-check procedures in healthcare settings to prevent medication errors and ensure patient safety.

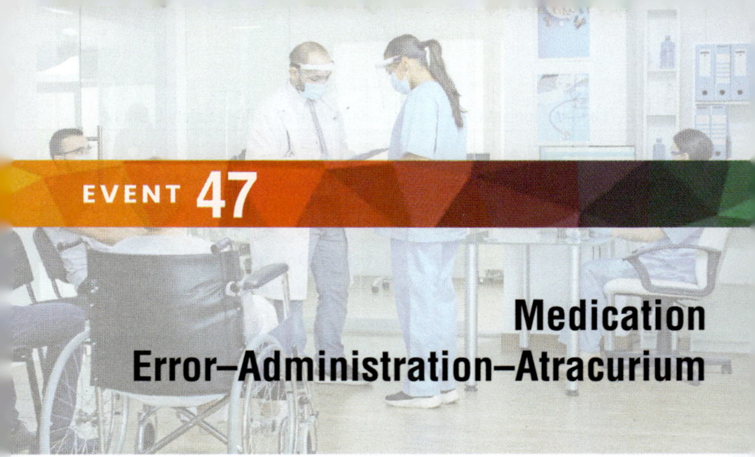

EVENT 47

Medication Error–Administration–Atracurium

EVENT NO.	PSE/047/092022
IPSG RELATED TO	IPSG 3 – Safe Handling of High-Risk Medication

CASE STUDY DESCRIPTION

An 8-year-old male child was admitted to PICU due to lung infection. Since the child was hemodynamically unstable, the treating team intubated the child and started their medical intervention. The child was responding well to the treatment process. On the fourth day, the child was hemodynamically stable and was planned for extubation. The child was extubated at 10:00 pm and was on an oxygen mask with 6 L/min. Around 12:30 am, the child developed respiratory distress, and the saturation dropped. The nursing team leader noticed the child's condition, and in hurry, she administered Inj. Atracurium 3 mg IV. Immediately, the child went into respiratory arrest. She presumed that the child was still intubated and therefore she administered Inj. Atracurium.

The nursing TL recognized her mistake and immediately called the duty doctor and re-intubated the child.

Positive Outcome

The child did not sustain any irreversible damage as the error was identified without delay and remedial action was taken.

Errors Encountered

- The TL administered muscle relaxant to the child who was already extubated.
- Inj. Atracurium was administered without doctor's order.

Lessons Learned

For nurse	For nurse educator	For nurse administrator
• Do not follow non-approved medication practices. • Always inform senior/duty doctor when patient condition deteriorates. • Regardless how experienced the nurses is, never circumvent two nurse verification for high-alert medication.	• Warn nurses during training that non-approved medication practices when normalized can lead to serious unintended harm. • Such scenarios can be discussed during training to sensitize nurses about safe practices, specially in critical care areas.	• Ensure safe staff ratios in high-risk areas. • Standing orders must be approved by medical head of the department, signed, printed and displayed for reference. • Ensure nurses follow two-Nurse verification for all high-alert medications.

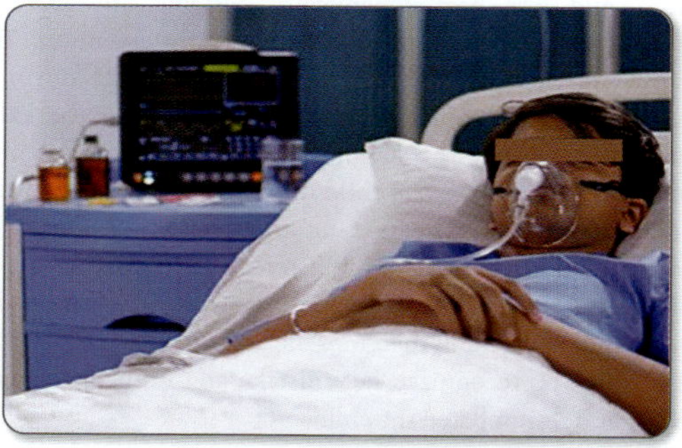

Figure 47 Standing orders improve patient care and increase nurse autonomy

Event-Based Learning Summary

In this instance, an 8-year-old male child was admitted to the Pediatric Intensive Care Unit (PICU) for a lung infection. The child had been responding well to the treatment but during the weaning process on day 4, after extubation, a critical situation unfolded. The child suddenly experienced respiratory distress and a drop in oxygen levels.

The Nursing Team Leader (TL) noticed the child's condition and, regrettably, presumed that the child was still intubated. Without adhering to standard operating procedures, the TL administered Inj. Atracurium 3 mg IV. This unfortunate incident highlights the necessity for healthcare professionals to be acutely aware of situations and remain extra vigilant. Administering high-alert medications should always be subject to stringent safety guidelines. In such cases, there is often no way to reverse a mistake, which underscores the crucial need for double-checking medications with another nurse. This incident serves as a stark reminder that some errors are irreversible, and it is the responsibility of healthcare providers to prioritize patient safety at all times.

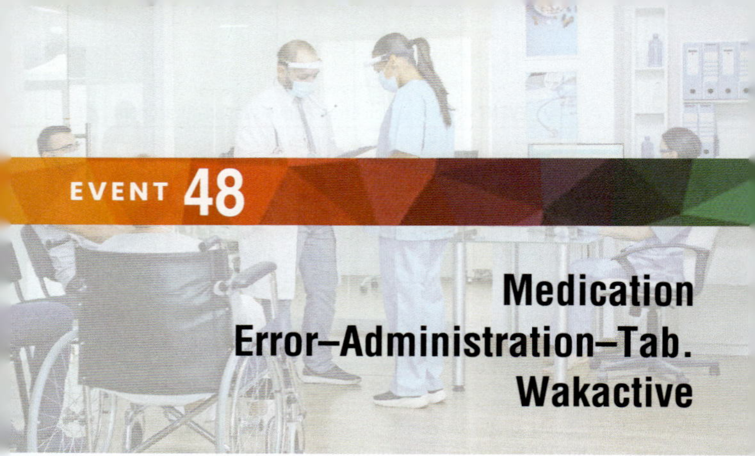

EVENT 48

Medication Error–Administration–Tab. Wakactive

EVENT NO.	PSE/048/092022
IPSG RELATED TO	None

CASE STUDY DESCRIPTION

A 45-year-old male patient with neurological dysfunction was admitted to a neuro ward with severe narcolepsy, and his surroundings utterly disoriented him. The treating team, on their rounds at 10:30 am, was informed about the patient's excessive daytime sleepiness by a patient attendant and the assigned staff. The treating team prescribed Tab. Wakactive 100 mg OD for the patient. The assigned staff indented Tab. Wakactive 200 mg (only 200 mg was available in the pharmacy) and missed the follow-up in her shift. During shift handover, she appraised that the drug was intended and yet to administer to the patient. The team leader received the prescription from the pharmacy at 4:00 pm and kept it in the receiving bay. The drug was unnoticed till 7:40 pm. At 7:58 pm, the assigned staff noticed that the Tab. Wakactive 100 mg was not administered to the patient. Immediately, she administered Tab. Wakactive 200 mg instead of 100 mg to the patient at 8:05 pm and documented in MAR sheet. The patient became restless, and the attendant informed the night TL for evaluation. During her assessment, it was found that Tab. Wakactive 200 mg was administered at 8:05 pm. Immediately, she explained the situation to the patient attendant and treating team about the medication error. The night TL acknowledged the mistake to the patient attendant and assured the same will not happen again.

Positive Outcomes

- The night TL intervened and understood the medication error and immediately explained the situation to the patient attendant and treating team.
- The error was self-reported.
- The night TL acknowledged the mistake to the patient attendant and assured the same will not happen again.

Errors Encountered

- The drug was not dispensed at the right time.
- The right strength of medication was not dispensed.
- After receiving it, the TL kept the drug in the bay without checking and intimating to the assigned staff.
- The assigned staff did not verify the order from the drug chart at the bedside before administration.

Lessons Learned

For nurse	For nurse educator	For nurse administrator
• Always ensure that nurse knows the medication that she is administering. • Always take the drug chart/file to the patient room to follow all rights during the medication administration.	When training nurses on medications, insist that nurses must make effort to learn about medication that are new to them.	• Medication management system can have a process to warn when medication strength ordered and available are not the same. • Appreciate when nurse are brave to admit their mistakes and apologize.

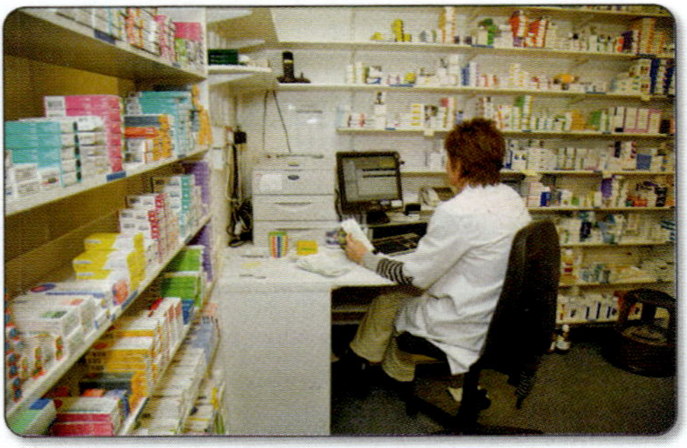

Figure 48 Dispensing medications from pharmacy

Event-Based Learning Summary

Nurses can draw valuable lessons from this event to enhance patient safety. It is crucial to double-check medications, clarify any prescription uncertainties, follow the five rights of medication administration (patient, medication, dosage, route, time), and maintain vigilance during high-occupancy or short-staffed situations. Thorough documentation, transparent reporting of errors, and educating patients about their medications are essential. Continuous learning to stay updated about medications is vital, and nurse leaders should provide guidance when less experienced staff are on duty. Additionally, always perform a final self-check before administering medications to ensure accuracy and patient well-being. Prioritizing these principles helps minimize the risk of medication errors and maintains a strong patient safety culture.

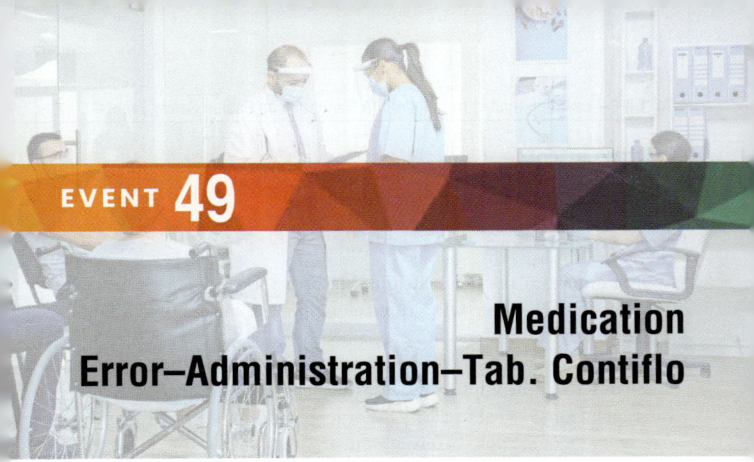

EVENT 49

Medication Error–Administration–Tab. Contiflo

EVENT NO.	PSE/049/092022
IPSG RELATED TO	None

CASE STUDY DESCRIPTION

The prescription for a 56-year-old male was Tab. Contiflo 2-2-1 OD in sequence. In the medication administration record sheet, it was transcribed as Tab. Contiflo 2-2-1 OD in sequence. The assigned nurse had concerns related to the order and clarified them with the treating consultant. The consultant repeated the order the same way he had prescribed it. The assigned nurse administered 2 tablets in the morning and in the afternoon. In the evening patients got shifted to the ward, the same medication handover was given to ward staff. And the ward staff administered the third dose, i.e., 1 tab at night. The next day, the order was transcribed in the same way. The consultant on rounds mentioned that since two tabs were given yesterday, administer only two tabs today to the assigned nurse. Alarmed by the consultant's statement, she immediately informed him that she had already administered two tabs in the morning. Now, the patient is due for an afternoon dose of 2 tabs since it is transcribed as 2-2-1, i.e., TDS. It was then realised that the order was misinterpreted as TDS dose where the medicine was to be administered as 2 tabs – Day 1, 2 tabs – Day 2, and 1 Tab- Day 3; The order written as 2-2-1 OD in sequence was understood as 2-2-1 (Three Times a day). The consultant withheld the medication till further order.

Positive Outcome

There was an attempt to clarify the order.

Errors Encountered

- Drug order was not prescribed in the correct format. 2-2-1 is usually a TDS dose. However, OD written alongside has created confusion.
- Strength of the drug was not prescribed.
- The nurse did not insist for new written order to clear the confusion. The order was incomplete and was not clear on the frequency.
- Assigned nurse failed to clarify the order with TL or the nurse manager to re-confirm the dose before administration.
- Failed to recognize that nurses are empowered NOT to administer medicine in case of ambiguous written orders.
- The same handover was given to another department nurse and caused the error to continue until consultant's, round the next day.

Lessons Learned

For nurse	For nurse educator	For nurse administrator
• Escalation to the seniors to be done in time—it can help prevent errors and provide an opportunity to promote patient safety. • A complete and correct written order must be requested from the doctors before executing the order. • Nurses must refer to the information available at the nursing units on medications.	• During nursing induction, CNEs, while dealing with medication management, the following points around written order must be emphasized: ▪ The order must be legible and complete (name, dose, route, frequency) ▪ Do not carry out orders with abbreviations which are not acceptable. ▪ If in doubt, first clarify with the doctor who ordered the medications • Training must be done for all those who are involved in the medication process, not just nurses.	• Insist and empower nurses not to carry out any orders that are not clearly understood. • Institute a process of nurse's reporting medication orders that are not compliant with hospital protocols. • Focus on orders that continue to use unacceptable/unsafe abbreviation. • Transcription of doctor's medication orders must be avoided. It is always recommended for doctors to order the medications directly on the medication chart.

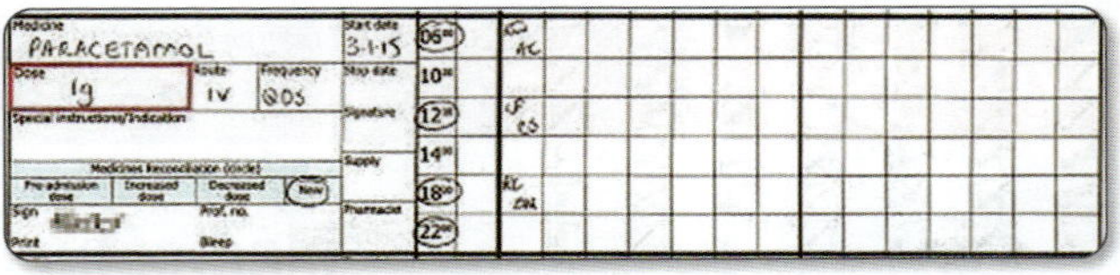

Figure 49 Sample of wrong prescription in MAR

Event-Based Learning Summary

The event underscores the importance of clear and unambiguous medication orders. Nurses should always seek clarification if an order appears unclear or incomplete. In this case, the misunderstanding of the prescription format led to a potential overdose. To prevent such errors, it is crucial to ensure that medication orders include all the necessary details: the drug name, dosage, route, frequency and duration. Additionally, nurses should feel empowered to withhold medication administration when orders are unclear or potentially harmful. Effective communication, especially when handing over patient care to another department, is essential to prevent errors from persisting.

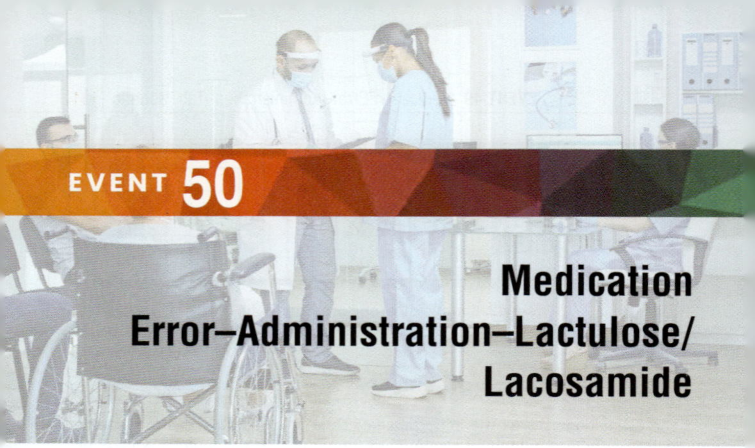

EVENT 50

Medication Error–Administration–Lactulose/ Lacosamide

EVENT NO.	PSE/050/092022
IPSG RELATED TO	None

CASE STUDY DESCRIPTION

A 60-year-old lady was admitted to the hospital with the chief complaints of slurred speech and quadriparesis. She was diagnosed with a cerebral stroke due to infarct. During the hospital stay, the patient complained of constipation, for which the consulting doctor advised Syrup Lactulose of 15 mL HS. The nurse indented Syrup Lacosamide (used for the treatment of seizures) instead of Syrup Lactulose. After receiving Syrup Lacosamide for two days the patient had increased blood pressure and involuntary movement of extremities. The patient's attendant informed that Syrup Lacosamide was not prescribed for the patient.

Positive Outcome

The patient attendant recognized the wrong medication.

Errors Encountered

- The nurse placed the wrong indent- Syrup Lacosamide instead of Lactulose.
- The patient received the wrong medication.
- The nurses failed to match the order with right medication.

- The nurses failed to identify the error themselves.
- During handover the nurses failed to check the medication.

Lessons Learned

For nurse	For nurse educator	For nurse administrator
• The nurse must be aware of LASA drugs during indent. • Always type in the full name of medication • Double check the indent before confirming on the system. • Never fail to do two self-checks matching the doctor's order and medicine available. • During shift handover at bedside both nurses must check the medications along with the orders.	• In-service education regarding look-alike and sound-alike drugs should be planned frequently, and evaluation should also be taken. • Such incident should be shared with all the nurses in a scenario-based session.	• Ensure the LASA drugs of the hospital is updated and displayed for all the nurse's units for reference. • Ensure HIS reflects alerts when LASA drugs are indented. • Ensure LASA drugs are labeled with stickers. • Conduct periodic audits for entire process of managing LASA drugs.

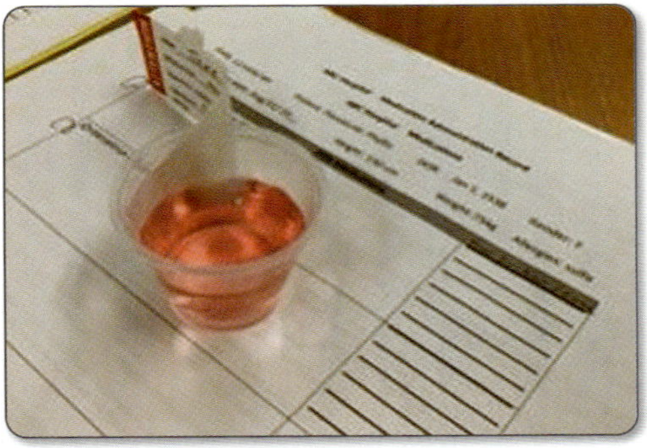

Figure 50 Cross checking the medication from MAR chart prior to administration

Event-Based Learning Summary

This event underscores the critical importance of thorough medication cross-checks and proper verification of administered drugs against the prescription, especially when dealing with LASA (Look-Alike, Sound-Alike) medications. Nurses must maintain unwavering vigilance in confirming the medication they are about to administer, particularly when faced with drugs that have similar names or appearances. In this case, the patient's relative played a pivotal role in identifying the error, highlighting the significance of providing patients and their families with clear education on the prescribed medications. The early recognition of the mistake and prompt intervention helped prevent more severe harm. Effective handovers and diligent medication checks by the assigned nurses are crucial steps in preventing such errors from occurring in the first place.

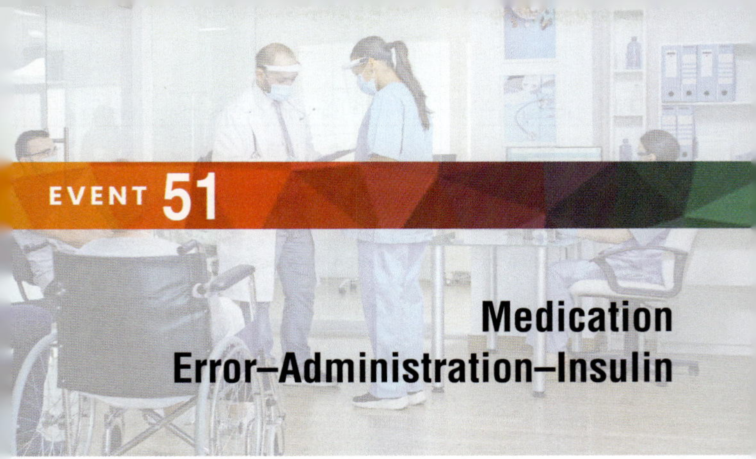

EVENT 51

Medication Error–Administration–Insulin

EVENT NO.	PSE/051/092022
IPSG RELATED TO	IPSG 3 – Safe Handling of High-Risk Medication

CASE STUDY DESCRIPTION

The nurse working in the ward was assigned to a diabetic patient. The doctor prescribed Human Mixtard 8 units subcutaneously. The nurse indented the same, double-checked with another nurse, and administered the drug. After a while, the patient complained of uneasiness and sweating. The RBS was checked immediately and it was 50 mg/dL.

Later it was identified that the nurse administered eight units of insulin from 100 IU/mL vial using a 40 units/mL tuberculin syringe instead of 100 units/mL tuberculin syringe.

Positive Outcome

The patient could be revived.

Errors Encountered

- The nurse missed to notice before indenting that the insulin prescribed was available in 2 forms 100 IU/1 mL and 40 IU/1 mL.
- The nurse used the wrong syringe for withdrawing the insulin.
- The double check did not include checking the right syringe.
- The dose of insulin injected was 2.5 times more than the actual prescribed dose.

Lessons Learned

For nurse	For nurse educator	For nurse administrator
• Nurses must be aware of different types of syringes and different strengths of insulin available in the hospital. • Double check of high alert medications should include checking the ampoules/vials against the order, amount drawn for the right patient. • The nurse must be extra vigilant about high-alert medication, specially common medication like insulin.	• Nurses must be trained on different types of syringes and different strengths of insulin available in the hospital. • Nurses must be provided hands-on training on such critical skills.	• Guidelines and policies for high alert medications on storage, prescription, dispensing, preparation, administration, monitoring, and documentation need to be defined. • The pharmacy and therapeutics committee can recommend having only one strength of Human Mixtard available in the hospital. The appropriate insulin syringe can also be standardized.

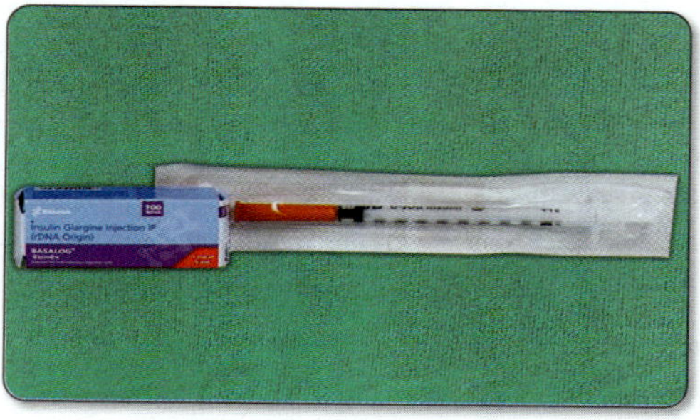

Figure 51 Administration of insulin with insulin syringe of same unit that is 100 IU/mL

Event-Based Learning Summary

In this medication error case, the critical lesson is the absolute necessity of diligent cross-checks and precise verification when dealing with insulin administration. Nurses should always be vigilant about the type of insulin prescribed, especially when it is available in multiple forms, such as 100 IU/10 mL and 40 IU/1 mL. Proper checks of the syringe being used are crucial, as this simple but significant error resulted in an insulin overdose putting the patient's health at risk. The importance of a thorough double-check process should be emphasized to ensure the safety of patients during medication administration. The nurse leader should focus on standardizing the syringe used for insulin administration, so as to eliminate the risk of nurses picking up the wrong syringe.

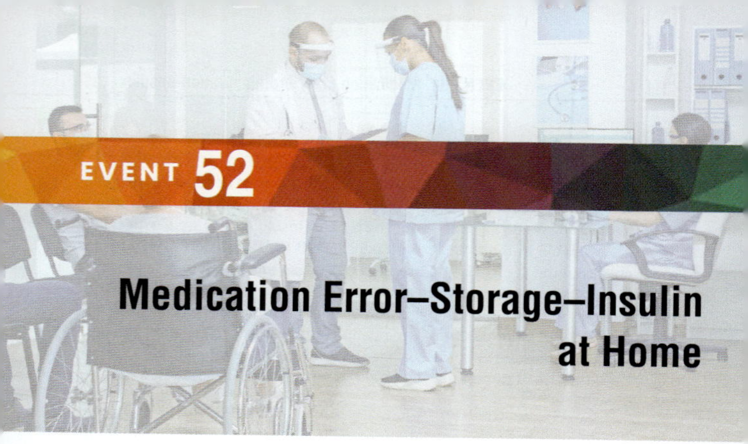

EVENT 52

Medication Error–Storage–Insulin at Home

EVENT NO.	PSE/052/092022
IPSG RELATED TO	None

CASE STUDY DESCRIPTION

A 50-year-old female patient got admitted on 02/10/2021 to the medical ward with complaints of increased fatigue, frequent urination, increased thirst, and weight loss of 10–15 kg. Blood investigations were done, which revealed (FBS-202 mg/dL, PPBS-415 mg/dL, and HbA1c-7.1%). The doctor diagnosed **Diabetes Mellitus**. The patient was treated with insulin therapy and oral medication for one week. CBG was monitored regularly. After stabilizing the blood glucose level, the patient was discharged with Insulin to be continued at home. The nurse gave discharge teaching, which included self-administration of Insulin, diet management, and follow-up care.

Re-admission: The patient, after 35 days (13/11/2021), came to EMS with complaints of giddiness, blurred vision, drowsiness, increased urination, and Insulin site ecchymosis. CBG was 495 mg/dL, and urine ketone was +ve.

The patient was started on treatment for Diabetic Ketoacidosis.

Patient history: On further communication with the patient and bystanders, it was found that the patient had kept the insulin at room temperature, and the same insulin syringe was used for one week.

Positive Outcomes

At the time of discharge, the nurse taught about:

- Self-administration of Insulin and oral medication (dosage, route, frequency).
- Dietary management regular follow-up.

Errors Encountered

- Storage of insulin was not taught to the patient at the time of discharge as per the manufacturer's recommendation.
- The patient was not informed about the warning signs of increased blood sugar.
- The patient was not informed regarding the change of the insulin syringe with each dose.

Lessons Learned

For nurse	For nurse educator	For nurse administrator
• Discharge education of a patient being sent home on Insulin must include the following: ■ Type of Insulin, dose and timing of Insulin ■ The storage of Insulin between use ■ Single use syringes, including the type of syringe ■ Recognizing symptoms of high and low blood sugar ■ What to do immediately in case of high and low blood sugar level ■ Where to reach for help ■ Importance of diet and physical activity. ■ The patient or patient attendant must be taught to withdraw the right dose of Insulin, in the right syringe at the right site and with the right technique. ■ A written demonstration must be taken before discharge.	• The nurses educator must design a short course on Diabetes Mellitus addressing all aspects of disease including- Insulin management, precautions around different type of Insulin, different types of Insulin syringes. • The course must also include the critical role of nurse in preventing complications related to low and high blood sugar, Insulin and what to do in an emergency.	• Plan, implement and evaluate the entire preparation and execution of training of nurses as mentioned in the columns of "For nurse" and "For Nurse Educators. • Implement periodic audits, on various aspects of nurses in the management of DM.

Contd...

For nurse	For nurse educator	For nurse administrator
• Always ensure that the patient and attendant have understood all teachings by using Teach-Back technique. • Self -administration of insulin can be initiated while in hospital to allow patient to have the confidence and experience.	• The role of nurses in patient education must be emphasized (refer to the points mentioned in the column " For Nurses).	

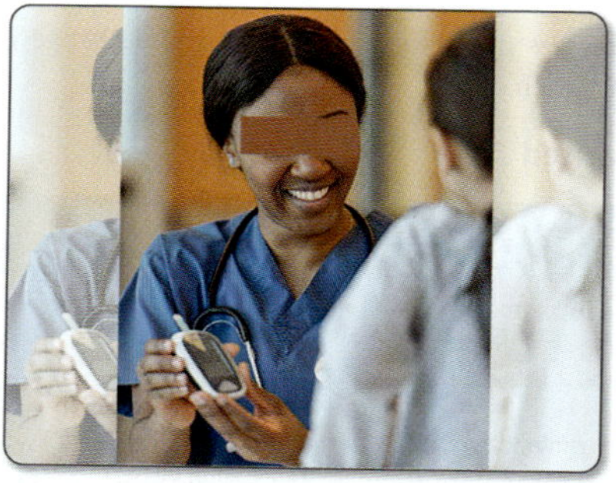

Figure 52 Nurse training the diabetic patient about glucometer

Event-Based Learning Summary

This case underscores the critical importance of robust patient education and effective communication, including the implementation of the "Teach-Back" technique. The patient's re-admission due to Diabetes Ketoacidosis highlights the need for comprehensive discharge instructions. The nurse correctly taught self-administration of insulin, dosage, dietary management, and the importance of regular follow-up. However, several crucial details were omitted from the teaching process. Storage instructions for insulin, in accordance with the manufacturer's recommendations, were not provided to the patient. Equally significant, the patient was not educated about the warning signs of increased blood sugar levels. Moreover, the importance of changing the insulin syringe with each dose was not adequately emphasized.

The "Teach-Back" technique, which involves asking patients to explain the instructions in their own words, could have helped ensure the patient's full comprehension. This approach enables healthcare providers to identify any areas of confusion or misunderstanding and provides an opportunity for clarification, ultimately promoting better patient self-management and reducing the risk of adverse events like re-admission for complications.

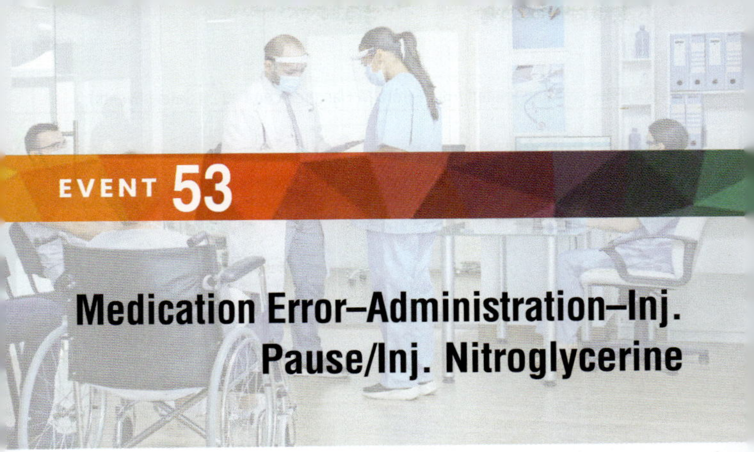

EVENT 53

Medication Error–Administration–Inj. Pause/Inj. Nitroglycerine

EVENT NO.	PSE/053/092022
IPSG RELATED TO	IPSG 3 – Safe Handling of High-Risk Medication

CASE STUDY DESCRIPTION

A male patient was admitted to the surgical ICU after a below-knee amputation. On the 4th POD, the patient developed bleeding from the surgical site. The doctor had ordered Inj. Pause (Tranexamic Acid), but the nurse brought Inj. Nitroglycerine from the drug cart. When the nurse was about to administer nitroglycerine, the senior nurse came and stopped it.

Positive Outcome

The nurses assessed the wound site and informed the doctor immediately.

Errors Encountered

- The nurse overlooked the LASA label in the Inj. Nitroglycerine.
- Inj. Pause and Inj. Nitroglycerine were not arranged as per LASA policy.
- The nurse failed to check the ampule.

Lessons Learned

For nurse	For nurse educator	For nurse administrator
• Three safety checks must be done by the nurse during the medication procedure. • Nurses must seek help if they are handling unfamiliar medications.	• Teaching and training staff on the significance and relevance of several stickers and color codes in the organization, e.g., color codes for high alert medication, LASA, etc. • In-service education regarding look-alike and sound-alike drugs should be planned frequently, and evaluation should also be taken.	• All nurses must be privileged for medication administration, ensuring that they are competent and follow safety practices. • Annual competency assessment to be introduced for medication administration.

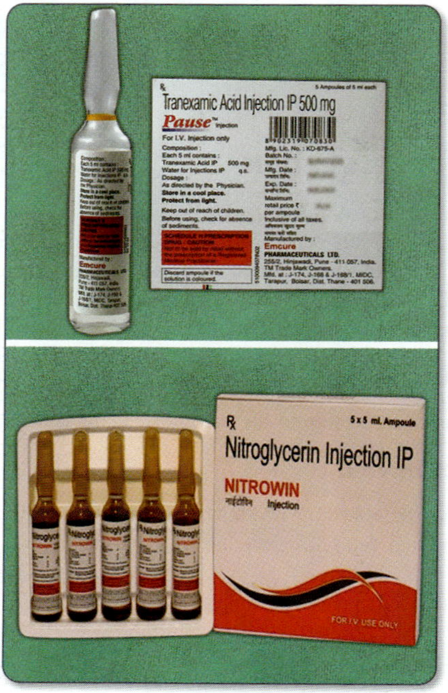

Figure 53 Injection pause and Inj. Nitroglycerine is a LASA drug (lookalike)

Event-Based Learning Summary

Nurses play a critical role in medication safety. Prioritize safe practices and vigilance to prevent errors. Adhere to LASA (Look-Alike, Sound-Alike) principles for correct medication administration. Use the five rights of medication as a checklist—right patient, right medication, right dose, right route and right time. Implement a self-triple check to ensure accuracy. Swiftly communicate concerns or discrepancies with healthcare providers. Patient safety depends on nurses' unwavering commitment to best practices during medication administration.

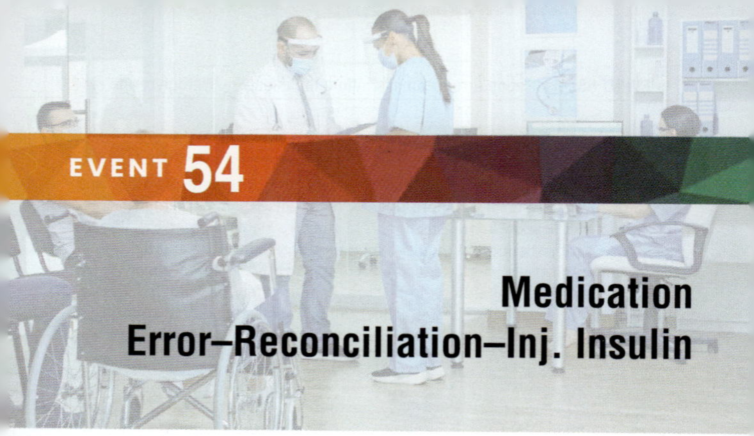

EVENT 54

Medication Error–Reconciliation–Inj. Insulin

EVENT NO.	PSE/054/092022
IPSG RELATED TO	None

CASE STUDY DESCRIPTION

A 75-year-old patient, a known case of DM for the past 20 years, was on Insulin Injection. He was posted for PTCA, and the Insulin order was withheld. Postprocedure, the patient was doing well, and the blood sugar was controlled with Insulin as ordered by the doctor. However, Insulin was missed in the discharge orders.

At home, the family members meticulously administered medications as per the doctor's discharge guidelines. His family checked his GRBS and found it in a higher range, but they ignored knowing that he had diabetes, until one day, when he was found unresponsive on his bed, he was rushed to the hospital.

Positive Outcome

The patient was saved.

Errors Encountered

- The doctor missed writing the insulin order in the discharge summary.
- The nurse also did not check whether the patient needed to be on insulin postprocedure.
- The family members also forgot to check on the insulin dose.

- There was no Teach-Back done to assess whether the family or patient understood the discharge guidelines.

Lessons Learned

For nurse	For nurse educator	For nurse administrator
• Teach-Back is necessary to confirm that the family understands the instructions provided. • Nurses can play a significant role by actively participating in medication reconciliation and review.	• Train nurses to involve patient and family members in the care as they could play a crucial role enlightening any gaps in the discharge medication and also gives an opportunity to clear their doubts. • Use simulated scenarios to emphasize the benefits of Teach-Back to ensure correct understanding of the education.	• Ensure the medication reconciliation of medication must be understood by all the nurses. • Must have a well-designed medication reconciliation form which can help in preventing such lapses.

Patient Information

First Name	Last Name	Date of Birth	ID
	Grey		ABC123
Community Pharmacy Name	**Community Pharmacy Number**	**Medication Management**	
		☑ Self-administration	☐ Caregiver Administration

Medication Allergies (Please state medication names and reactions you get)
N/A

Medication Information Obtained From (Select all that applies)
☑ Patient Interview ☑ Family/Caregiver Interview
☐ Specialist Letter ☐ Admission Medication Reconciliation
☐ EHR/EMR ☐ Discharge Medication Order Form
☑ Pharmacy ☐ Outside Facility Medication List
☑ Medication Vials/Boxes ☑ Patient's Own Medication List
☐ Blister Packs ☐ Other:

Best Possible Medication History BPMH Completed By: Date: 16.12.2022

Medication Name	Dose	Route	Frequency	Indication	Prescribed By	Discrepancy	Resolution Plan	Action
Metoprolol	95mg	Oral	Twice Daily	Hypertension	Dr	☐	New Medication	Start
Alendronate	60mg	Oral	Once Weekly	Osteoporosis	Dr	☐		Continue
Calcium Carbonate	250mg	Oral	Twice Daily	Osteoporosis	Dr	☐		Continue
Acetaminophen	300mg	Oral	4x daily	Osteoarthritis -02/2022	Dr	☑	Dose change	Stop
Ibuprofen	500mg	Oral	Twice Daily	Osteoarthritis - 11/2021	Dr	☑	Switch to Tylenol only	Stop
Aspirin	300mg	Oral	Daily	Heart protection -hypertension	Dr	☑		Continue
Felodipine	2.5mg	Oral	Daily	Hypertension	Dr	☑	Switch to Metoprolol	Stop
Lisinopril	35mg	Oral	Daily	Kidney protection -hypertension	Dr	☐	Switch to Amlodipine	Stop
Amlodipine	10mg	Oral	Daily	Kidney protection -hypertension, 10/2022	Dr	☐	New Medication	Start
Metolazone	5mg	Oral	Daily	Diuretic- hypertension- 10/2022	Dr	☐	New Medication	Start
Acetaminophen	500mg	Oral	4x Daily	Osteoarthritis -12/2022 update	Dr	☐	New dosage	Start

Figure 54 Filled medication reconciliation form

Event-Based Learning Summary

Medication reconciliation during discharge is a crucial step in ensuring patient safety. Healthcare providers, including doctors and nurses, must be diligent in reviewing and accurately documenting all medications a patient should continue postprocedure or upon returning home. Clear communication with the patient and the family regarding medication regimens, especially for chronic conditions like diabetes, is essential. A "check-back" process (Teach-Back) should be in place to assess the patient and family's understanding of post-discharge medication instructions. This vigilance can prevent serious health crises and hospital readmissions due to missed medications.

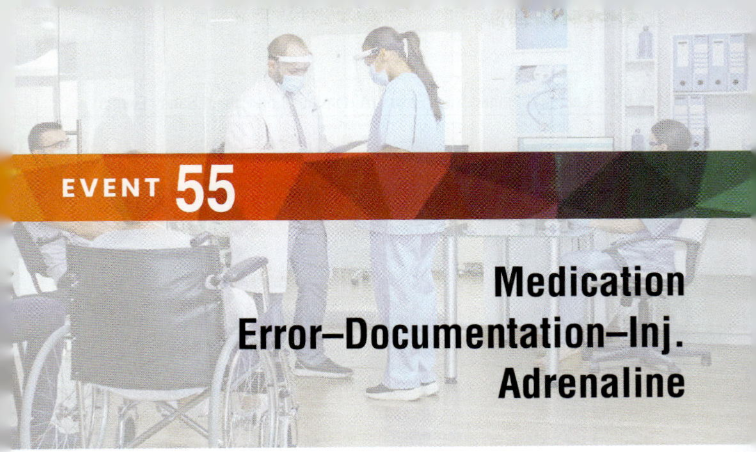

EVENT 55

Medication Error–Documentation–Inj. Adrenaline

EVENT NO.	PSE/055/092022
IPSG RELATED TO	IPSG 3 – Safe Handling of High-Risk Medication

CASE STUDY DESCRIPTION

A newborn baby was admitted to the neonatal ICU with the diagnosis of preterm/RDS on 07/08/2021. The baby developed desaturation and bradycardia. Pediatrician ordered giving Inj. Adrenaline 0.1 mg IV stat and medication was administered at 10:30 pm, but the assigned staff had not done the double check and neither was it documented.

Positive Outcome

The documentation error was identified by the senior nurse.

Errors Encountered

- High-alert medication was not double checked.
- Documentation was also not done.

Lessons Learned

For nurse	For nurse educator	For nurse administrator
• Always have another nurse to check the rights of high-alert medication. • Remember to document the medication immediately after the administration. But in case of an emergency situation document soon after the situation is stabilized.	• Ensure all staff must have adequate orientation to safe and timely documentation. • CNEs should be organized periodically to refresh their medication safety and patient safety knowledge.	• Ensure senior nurses are available to mentor fresh graduate nurses and provide effective supervision. • Audits of medication chart must be done frequently.

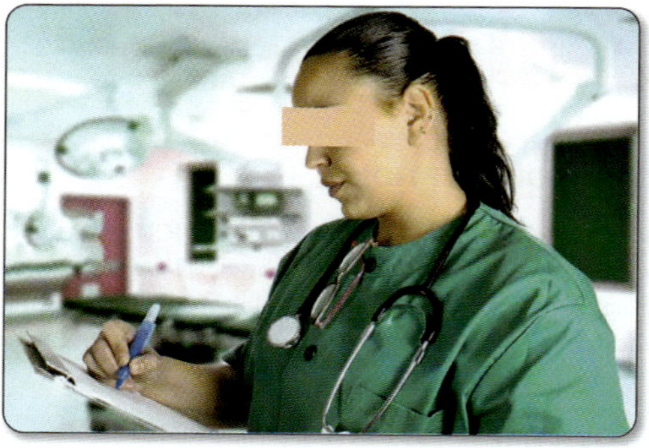

Figure 55 Clinical documentation by nurse

Event-Based Learning Summary

Accurate and timely documentation is crucial in healthcare, especially for high-alert medications. Even during critical situations, it is vital to ensure that medications are properly documented to maintain a complete record of patient care. In cases where multiple healthcare providers are involved, a double-check process should be established to prevent documentation oversights. Nurses, particularly those in training, should be educated about the protocols and importance of documenting all aspects of patient care.

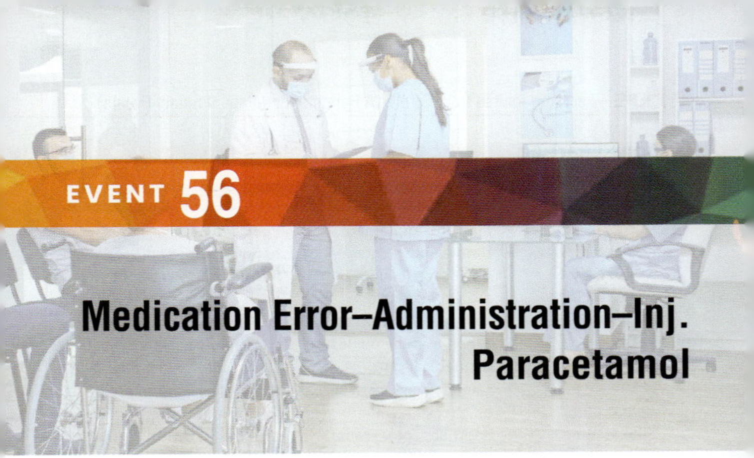

EVENT 56

Medication Error–Administration–Inj. Paracetamol

EVENT NO.	PSE/056/092022
IPSG RELATED TO	None

CASE STUDY DESCRIPTION

A 2-year-old child was admitted with fever to the adult ward as there were no beds in the pediatric department. The prescription was to administer 200 mg of Inj. Paracetamol 8-hourly. The assigned nurse connected the injection paracetamol (1000 mg in 100 mL) through the infusion pump and went to her other patients. After one hour, when she returned to check, it was found that the whole 1 gram of Inj. Paracetamol was completed. Immediately it was escalated to the treating doctor, and the patient was given the antidote (Acetylcysteine).

Positive Outcome

Immediate escalation of the error saved the child from complications of overdose.

Errors Encountered

- The selection of the pump was wrong.
- The child was admitted to an adult ward, where nurses are used to adult doses. These nurses do not have pediatric competencies.
- The patient received an overdose of Paracetamol.

Lessons Learned

For nurse	For nurse educator	For nurse administrator
• Nurses to always check with another nurse for any orders that are not clear to them. Better to SPEAK UP and clear doubts than assume. • Use the syringe pumps for pediatric doses.	• Plan and implement training of selected nurses from adult area in pediatric competencies. • When training nurses on medication safety always insist on checking with another senior nurse of any medication or doses. • The training must include the drug calculations for pediatric doses.	• Pediatric cases are to be handled only by nurses having age-related competencies. • Only nurses having those special privileges to administer medications. • Identifying 'backup area' for pediatric admissions in case of spillovers. • Diluting of medications in 'backup area' to be done by senior nurses only.

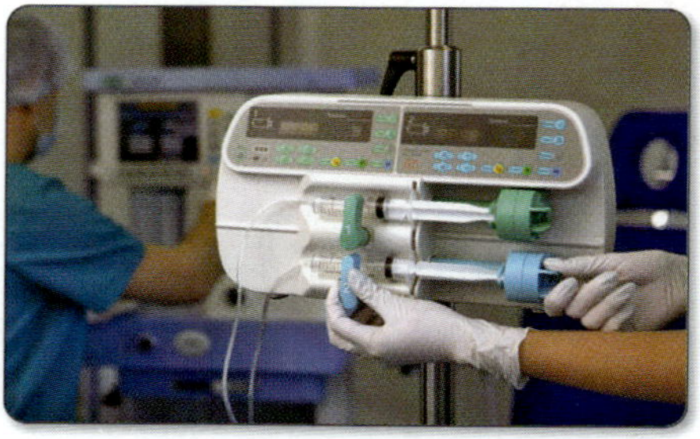

Figure 56 Administration of medication to pediatric patient through syringe pump

Event-Based Learning Summary

When dealing with pediatric patients, it is essential to ensure that healthcare providers have the necessary pediatric competencies. Medication administration for children requires precise calculations and the use of appropriate equipment, such as syringe pumps, to control the dosage accurately. Pediatric patients may be more sensitive to medication errors; so, nurses and healthcare teams should exercise extra caution and closely monitor them, particularly during medication administration. Regular competency training for nurses and ensuring access to pediatric-specific medications and equipment in adult wards can help prevent such errors. Furthermore, maintaining open lines of communication between healthcare providers is vital for prompt error detection and resolution.

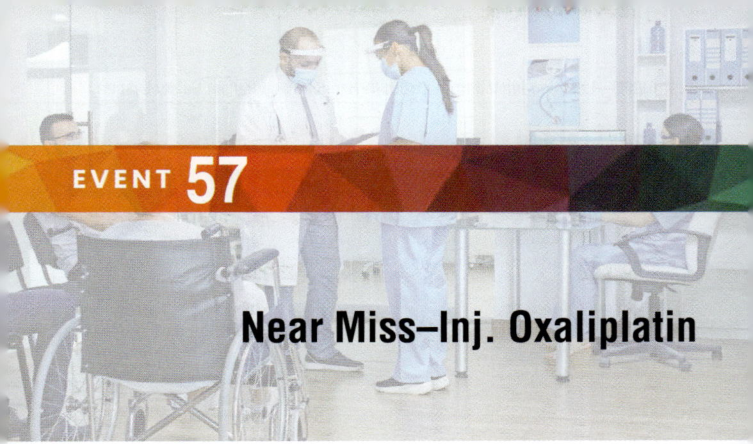

EVENT 57

Near Miss–Inj. Oxaliplatin

EVENT NO.	PSE/057/092022
IPSG RELATED TO	None

CASE STUDY DESCRIPTION

A 55-year-old male patient was admitted to the hospital in Hemato-oncology ward. He was on Inj. Oxaliplatin IV 120 mg. The dose was changed from 120 mg to 100 mg. The changed dose was not transcribed to chemo orders. Hence 120 mg was intended. However, the error was identified before the dilution of the medication.

Positive Outcome

Since the error was caught before dilution of drug, the patient received the correct dose.

Error Encountered

Transcription error.

Lessons Learned

For nurse	For nurse educator	For nurse administrator
• Check and recheck the doctor's orders if the doctors are not writing directly into the medication chart. • All chemo drugs must be double checked with another nurse.	Training and privileging of all nurses involved in handling chemo drugs.	The nurse administrator must work with the senior management to have the policy of medication orders to be written in the MAR chart directly by the doctors.

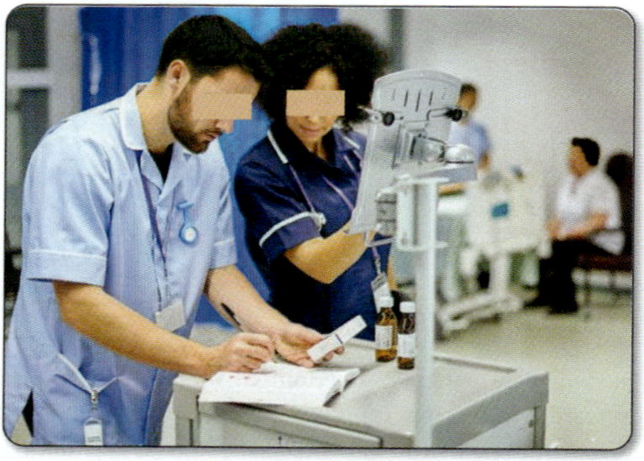

Figure 57 Checking and rechecking the chemotherapeutic medication as per doctor's order to avoid medication error

Event-Based Learning Summary

Near-miss incidents, particularly involving chemotherapy drugs like Oxaliplatin with a narrow therapeutic range, underscore the critical need for precision and vigilance in healthcare. Medication transcription errors can lead to severe consequences. It is essential for healthcare professionals to prioritize patient safety by double-checking and confirming all medication orders, especially in the case of chemotherapy drugs with a narrow therapeutic range. Taking shortcuts should never be an option, and healthcare providers should never hesitate to ask for assistance when in doubt, minimizing the risk of potentially harmful errors. It is always safer to avoid transcribing the drug orders from the order sheet. It is always safe to get the doctors to write or to prescribe directly into MAR sheet.

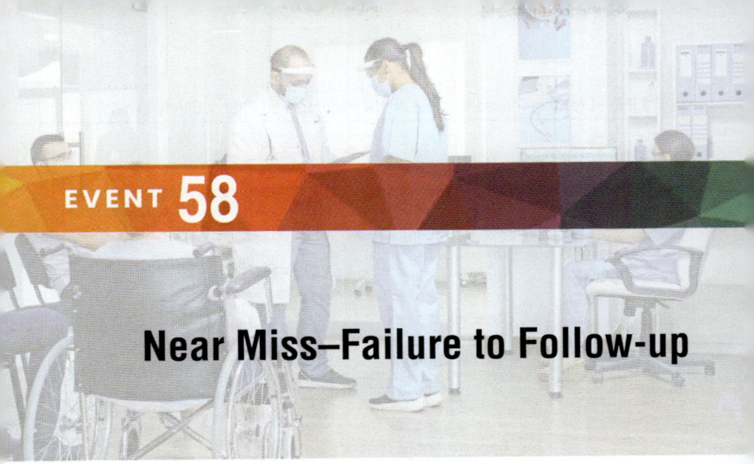

EVENT 58

Near Miss–Failure to Follow-up

EVENT NO.	PSE/058/092022
IPSG RELATED TO	None

CASE STUDY DESCRIPTION

A 35-year-old male patient was brought to ER with complaints of severe abdominal pain, vomiting and not passing stools for two days. The patient had tachycardia, tachypnea, hypotension, restlessness, and abdominal distention on examination. A baseline investigations were sent, IV fluids started, patient was kept NPO, and CT abdomen was done. The patient was transferred to the ward following an hour after the CT, the patient's condition deteriorated in the ward. Later the patient was diagnosed with intestinal obstruction.

Positive Outcome

The patient assessment and initiation of treatment and investigations including CT scan was done without delay.

Errors Encountered

- The radiology department did not report the critical finding.
- The nurses also failed to follow-up the CT report.

Lessons Learned

For nurse	For nurse educator	For nurse administrator
Nurses must act proactively to collect critical report to ensure timely intervention so that patient prognosis can be better.	When training nurses on policy of critical alert reporting, the educator can emphasize the need for nurses to be on alert to follow the critical reports of stat investigations, rather than waiting for the department to report.	• The organization must define a policy on critical result reporting. • Periodic audits on critical value reporting process to ensure compliance. • The nursing administrator to have multi-departmental discussion when such lapses happen.

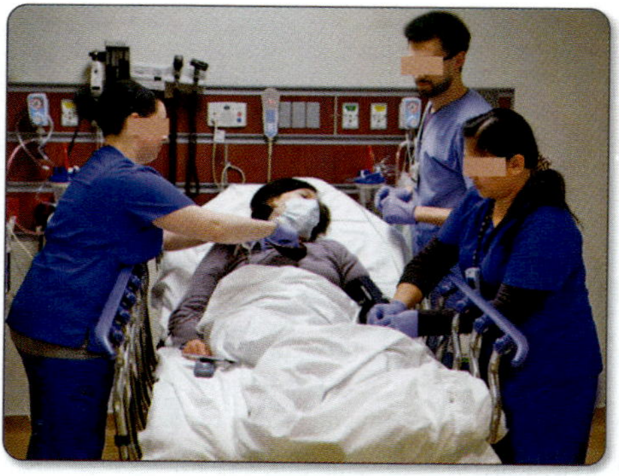

Figure 58 Intensive patient assessment

Event-Based Learning Summary

While timely assessments and interventions play a vital role in patient care, following up on crucial test results is equally critical. In situations involving high-risk conditions like intestinal obstruction, a delay in obtaining diagnostic results can gravely impact patient outcomes. Given the narrow margins for error, it is essential that healthcare professionals do not rely solely on one department for critical updates. Regular proactive follow-ups, particularly when a patient's condition can change rapidly, are paramount. Ensuring clear communication channels between departments and having protocols in place for immediate reporting of critical values can prevent such near misses. Every healthcare professional should prioritize following through on their patient's care, especially in a busy environment. When in doubt or overwhelmed, seeking help or confirmation can make all the difference.

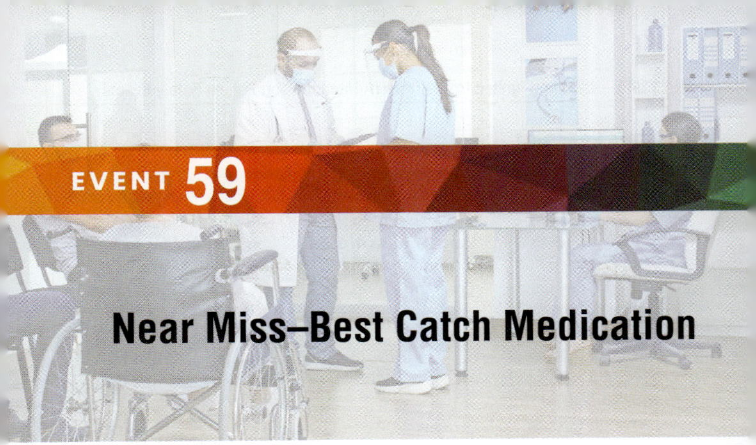

EVENT 59

Near Miss–Best Catch Medication

EVENT NO.	PSE/059/092022
IPSG RELATED TO	None

CASE STUDY DESCRIPTION

The patient was admitted on 29th June and was posted for right inguinal hernia repair (Meshplasty) on 30th June 2022. During her initial nursing assessment, the assigned staff nurse identified that the patient who was posted for surgery the next day was still taking his routine antiplatelet drug Tab. Ticaspan 90 mg. She immediately informed the on-duty Resident Medical Officer (RMO) and the consultant about the same. The patient's surgery was rescheduled, and he was discharged on the same day.

Positive Outcomes

- The nurse identified the drug as an antiplatelet drug
- Another reason for this 'Best Catch' was the nursing department's initiative of encouraging nurses to study the prescribed drugs of their assigned patients.

Errors Encountered

Error prevented.

Lessons Learned

For nurse	For nurse educator	For nurse administrator
• Nurses must thoroughly verify medical orders/ prescriptions before executing them. • Nurses must have sound knowledge about the drugs that they administer. This can be the safety net for many such incidents.	Include such "Best Catch" events in CNEs or during training programs for nurses.	Institute recognition and rewards for such "Best Catch" events. This will promote nurses to be vigilant to such oversights which could lead to patient harm.

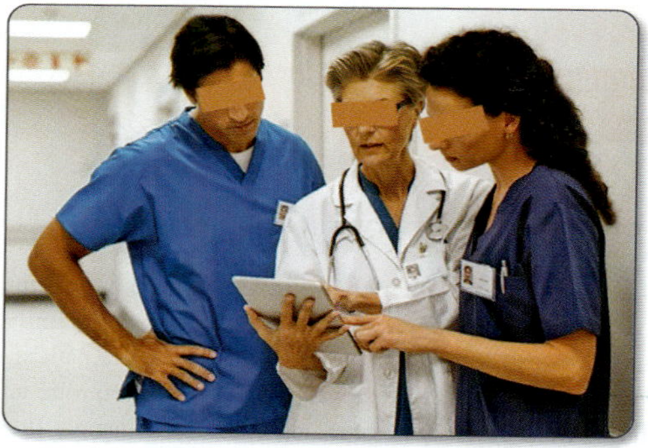

Figure 59 Nurses cross checking the orders with the doctor

Event-Based Learning Summary

This near miss highlights the importance of thorough medication reconciliation and knowledge of a patient's drug regimen, especially when surgical procedures are involved. Nurses play a crucial role in catching potential medication errors, and their vigilance can prevent adverse events. Encouraging nurses to actively study prescribed medications, ask questions, and verify the patient's drug history are some of the effective strategies to enhance patient safety. In busy healthcare settings, these practices should be routine to ensure the well-being of the patients, even if it results in procedure rescheduling, as patient safety should always take precedence.

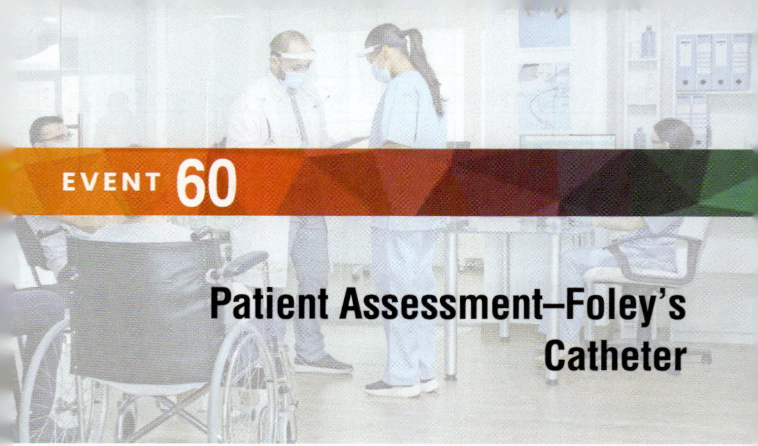

EVENT 60

Patient Assessment–Foley's Catheter

EVENT NO.	PSE/060/092022
IPSG RELATED TO	None

CASE STUDY DESCRIPTION

A 38-year-old male had been admitted to Spinal Cord Injury unit after sustaining fractures of thoracic vertebrae (6 & 7) due to fall from height. The patient had no sensory or motor function below D6.

The patient was on an indwelling urinary catheter. One day when the staff nurse went to check the vital signs noticed that he had profuse sweating and was complaining about severe headache and chest pain. His heart rate was 62/min, and his blood pressure at that time was 180/110 mm Hg. When she went to the nurse's station to inform the concerned doctor, she also reported to the nurse in-charge. The in-charge nurse on assessment noticed that the patient's bladder was distended. She immediately examined the urinary drainage system and noticed a kink in the catheter; the urine was not draining. Immediately she released the kink, and the urine started draining. The patient became stable within the next 10 minutes (BP: 140/90 mm Hg). The doctor on telephonic consultation said that it is a typical episode of autonomic dysreflexia and had advised giving Tab. Nifedipine 5 mg sublingually if diastolic BP is above 100 mm Hg. But it was not given as his blood pressure had stabilized within 10 minutes.

Positive Outcomes

- The nurse reached patient's bedside at the right time.
- The timely assessment and physical examination skills of in-charge nurse saved the patient from further harm.

Errors Encountered

The kink and urinary retention was not noticed by the assigned nurse.

Lessons Learned

For nurse	For nurse educator	For nurse administrator
• The nurse should check free flow of urine whenever they are at the bedside, specially in patients who have sensory loss. • When assigned to patients with diagnosis that the nurse is not familiar ask for guidance and supervision, and when in doubt escalate without any delay.	• The nurse educators should plan and conduct trainings for patients with uncommon diagnosis. • Such events can be made part of trainings through simulation-based scenarios.	The nurse administrator should be alert to ensure supervision by experienced nurses when patients are admitted with uncommon diagnosis.

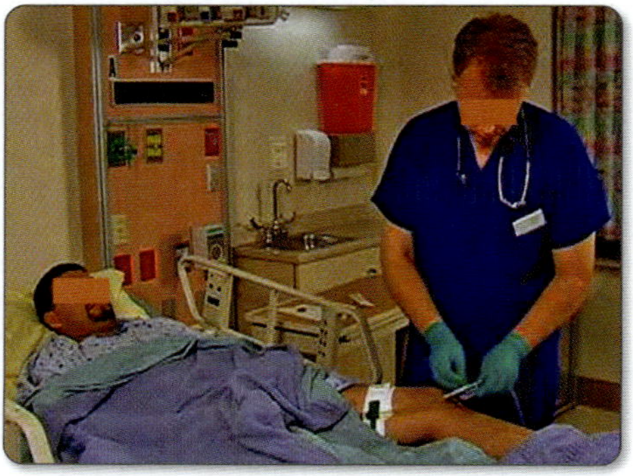

Figure 60 Nurse ensures there is no kink in the catheter and urobag to promote free flow of urine

Event-Based Learning Summary

This case emphasizes the importance of thorough and frequent patient assessment, especially in individuals with spinal cord injuries. Autonomic dysreflexia is a life-threatening condition that can occur in such patients. Nurses must be vigilant in monitoring patients with spinal cord injuries for potential signs and symptoms, such as hypertension, headache or chest pain. In this case, prompt assessment and action by the in-charge nurse led to the resolution of the issue. However, the initial oversight of not checking the urinary catheter for proper drainage is a critical reminder that the urinary system must be continuously monitored to prevent complications like autonomic dysreflexia. Nurses should be aware of the risks and signs of autonomic dysreflexia as early intervention is essential for patient safety.

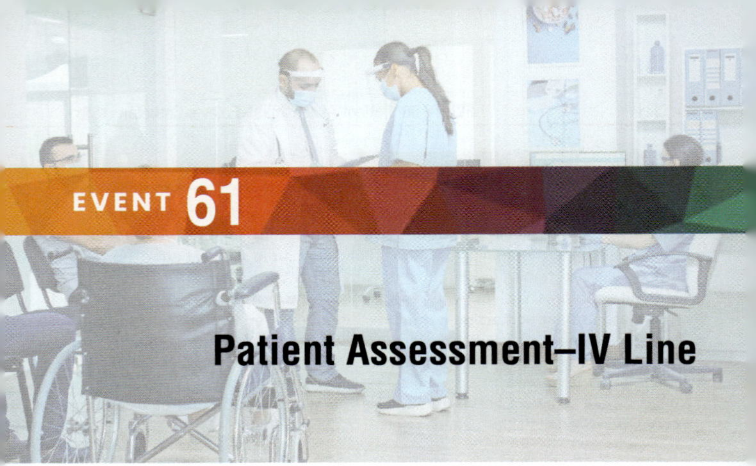

EVENT 61

Patient Assessment–IV Line

EVENT NO.	PSE/061/092022
IPSG RELATED TO	None

CASE STUDY DESCRIPTION

A 19-year-old boy was admitted to the orthopedic ward with a fracture of the left femur and left radius after a road traffic accident. On the 3rd postoperative day, the peripheral IV line had to be changed as the existing one was not patent. Inj. Cloxacillin and Inj. Crystalline Penicillin were due to be administered at 11 pm. The nurse forgot to start a new IV access in her busy work schedule. She realized it only after loading the injections for administration.

A new line was inserted at the antecubital fossa at 11:30 pm; the loaded injections were administered soon after with a three-way extension. Immediately after administering the injections, 300 mL of whole blood was connected. The nurse returned after 5 minutes to check the vital signs and realized that the blood was not flowing; instead, the blood bag was filled with bright red blood as the IV cannula was in the artery. The blood from the patient had flown into the blood bag, not vice versa. The peripheral line was removed immediately. The following day, the hand worsened due to lack of blood supply and became gangrenous. A consultation was taken with a vascular surgeon after 12 hours. Inj. Heparin infusion was started. However, the gangrene in the hand remained the same. The doctor had to wait for demarcation and amputate the patient's fingers to the intermediate phalanges.

Positive Outcome

None.

Errors Encountered

- The flashback of arterial blood was not noticed as the nurse had occluded the line with pressure. The loaded Inj. Cloxacillin and Crystalline Penicillin were given and secured with a three-way extension.
- She failed to notice the bright red artery blood in the extension line while she started the blood transfusion.
- The nurse went deeper into the antecubital fossa and accidentally cannulated the artery instead of the vein.
    - Adequate light was not there when the IV line was initiated.
- Failed to escalate such serious event to the consultant which led to delay of 12 hours in starting Inj. Heparin.

Lessons Learned

For nurses	For nurse trainer	For nurse administrator
• Ensure there is adequate light when performing any procedure. • Be alert in observing patient and his response while performing even common procedure. • If doubtful in performing any procedure take help from senior staff.	• When training nurses on common procedure include what can go wrong and how to avoid them. • Include such incidents in training to emphasize the need for nurses to be diligent even in common procedures like IV cannulation. • During the training of blood transfusion protocol insist on two-person verification at the bedside (if this was practiced may be the second nurse might have noticed the IV cannula being in an artery).	• Address the root cause of the failure to escalate. This may involve addressing issues such as lack of resources, a culture of fear or intimidation, or inadequate training. • Implement corrective actions. This may involve changes to policies, procedures, or protocols, additional staff education and training, or other interventions as appropriate.

Note

Legal implications- Since the patient's fingers had to be amputated there is cause that effect relationship. This case is highly liable for a law suit where the nurse can be charged with negligence resulting in award of huge compensation.

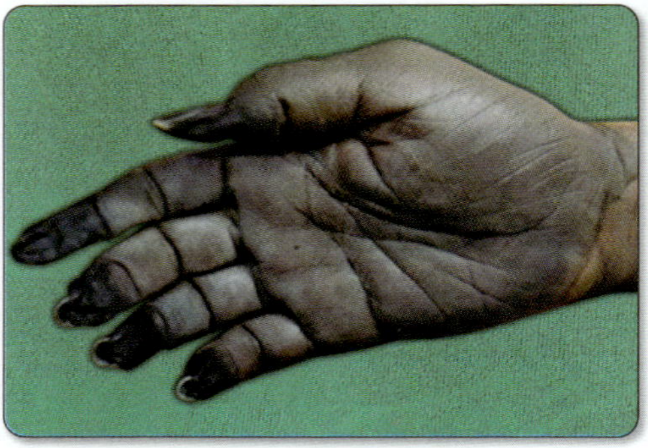

Figure 61 Gangrene showing clear line of demarcation

Event-Based Learning Summary

This incident underscores the critical importance of meticulous IV-line management and careful administration of medications. Nurses should never rush when inserting IV lines and should always ensure they are in the appropriate vein, especially when dealing with multiple tasks. Inadequate lighting and rushing can lead to errors like the one in this case, where an artery was mistakenly cannulated instead of a vein. Additionally, early intervention and expert consultation are vital when such errors occur. This case highlights the severe consequences of such mistakes as drug administration into an artery can result in acute arterial spasm, tissue damage, and in extreme cases, gangrene. It serves as a stark reminder of the need for vigilance and diligence in clinical practice to prevent life-threatening complications, even while performing common procedures.

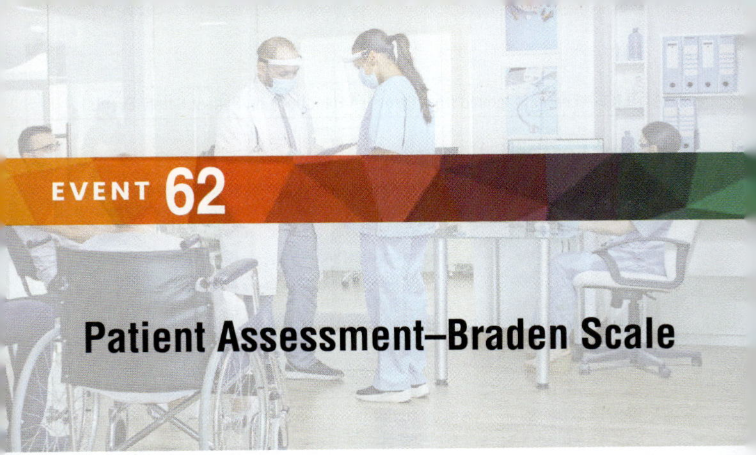

EVENT 62

Patient Assessment–Braden Scale

EVENT NO.	PSE/062/092022
IPSG RELATED TO	None

CASE STUDY DESCRIPTION

A 65-year-old woman was admitted to the hospital to get treatment for a fracture of right tibia and fibula. The patient underwent an intramedullary nailing procedure. In the postoperative period, the admitting nurse assessed and gave a score of 14 according to the Braden scale. But the air mattress and protocol were not followed. The second postoperative day skin Braden assessment score was 20 and third postoperative day the night nurse reported the presence of discolored intact skin on sacrum then finally, the patient was placed on an air mattress. On fifth day, the patient was discharged to a local skilled nursing facility, where he was diagnosed with stage IV decubitus ulcer.

Positive Outcome

None.

Errors Encountered

- Wrong Braden scale assessment.
- Failure to assess the skin and identify skin changes.
- Failure to implement preventive nursing interventions.

Lessons Learned

For nurse	For nurse educator	For nurse administrator
• The nurses must do the Braden scale assessment diligently with the purpose of understanding the risk level of the patient. • Along with Barden scale skin assessment of pressure injury risk points must also be done. • Assigned nurses must be proactive in initiating the preventive measures (appropriate skin care, repositioning, and appropriate air mattress). • Seek help from seniors to plan the nursing care, do not forget to seek help while repositioning the patient. • Raise incident report as soon as nurse finds any skin changes on pressure points.	• Have a comprehensive pressure injury prevention and management workshop for all the nurses working with vulnerable category of patients. • Train and re-train on importance of skin assessment, principles of prevention and management. • Provide hands-on training on lifting, turning and positioning the patient on bed. • Provide ongoing education and support to nurses to ensure that they are up-to-date on the latest research and best practices related to pressure ulcer prevention and management. • Sensitize all cadre of nurses on hospital acquired pressure injury being one of the most critical nursing sensitive quality indicators. Also educate nurses on the risk of hospital getting into malpractice suit in which nurses also will be held accountable.	• Institute a pressure injury prevention program which detail resources required, preventive and management protocols and outcome indicators. • Institute pressure injury prevalence audits and regular Braden and skin assessment of vulnerable patients by a senior nurse at-least once in a day. • While doing root cause analysis focus on shortage of resources, the reason for deviation from laid out protocols. Involve the front line nurses in these discussions so that the problems from the bedside can be heard and addressed.

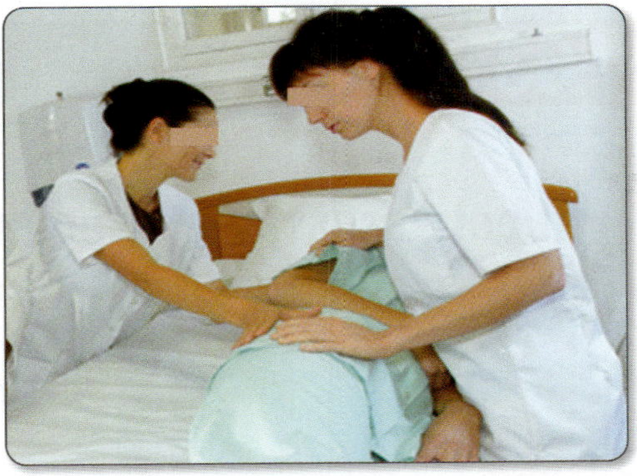

Figure 62 Nurses changing the position and providing back care two hourly

Event-Based Learning Summary

This case highlights the critical importance of diligent skin assessment and preventive measures while caring for immobilized or postoperative patients. Nurses must follow established protocols for maintaining skin integrity, including the use of pressure-relieving devices such as air mattresses. Failure to follow these protocols can result in serious pressure ulcers and potential legal repercussions. Proper assessment and documentation are essential in ensuring that the patient's condition is accurately monitored and that appropriate interventions are implemented to prevent complications like pressure ulcers. This case underscores the need for nurses to be vigilant in adhering to preventive measures and thorough documentation to protect patients and mitigate legal risks.

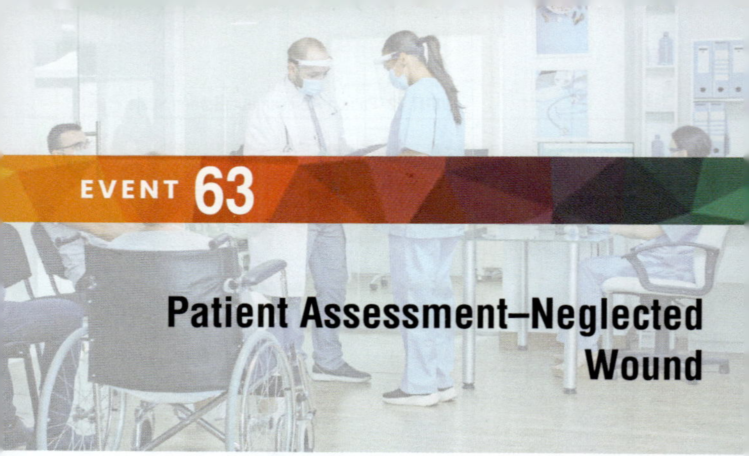

EVENT 63

Patient Assessment–Neglected Wound

EVENT NO.	PSE/063/092022
IPSG RELATED TO	None

CASE STUDY DESCRIPTION

Mr Ram, a 50-year-old was admitted with severe traumatic brain injury, low sensorium, acute kidney injury (AKI), Right Clavicle Fracture and cervical injury with tracheostomy and arm sling. The senior nursing supervisor asked the assigned nurse to remove the collar to assess the skin under the collar. The senior nurse was shocked to see the sore in the cervical region. On asking the assigned nurse, she came to know that collar was not removed since 3 days. The doctor was informed and advised to apply soft roll sling and T-Bact ointment.

Positive Outcomes

- Effective supervision by nursing supervisor by assessing the patient herself.
- There was a policy for provision of cervical collar care.

Errors Encountered

- Failure to assess skin under the collar for 3 days.
- Failure to provide collar care for 3 days.
- Incomplete handing over at the bedside.

Lessons Learned

For nurse	For nurse educator	For nurse administrator
• Periodical assessment and collar care to be followed as per hospital protocol. • Focus on bedside handover in every shift wherein two nurses check the skin of all vulnerable sites. • Involve patient and companion in the care.	• Train all nurses on skin care for patient on cervical collar and other such immobilizing devices. • Train them also on application of such devices. • These training sessions are effective if they are conducted as hands-on training.	• Monitor compliance to cervical collar care policies and procedures. • Conduct regular competency assessments. • Ensure interdisciplinary collaboration. • Institute skin injury prevalence audits for patients on immobilizing devices and ensure such patients are assisted by a senior nurse at-least once in a day.

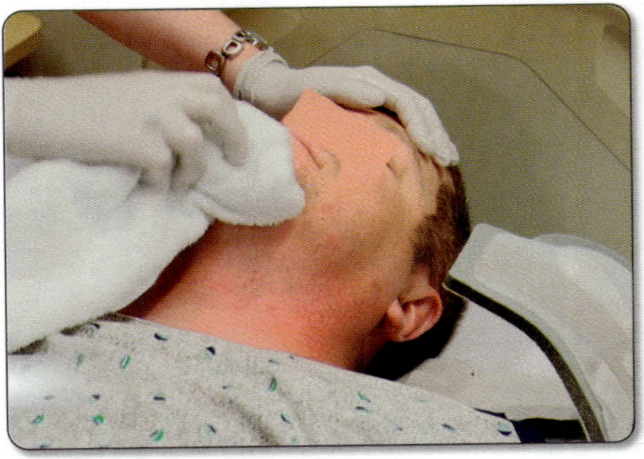

Figure 63 Cervical collar care

Event-Based Learning Summary

This case underscores the importance of diligent nursing care, especially when dealing with immobilized or critically ill patients. Cervical collar care, regular skin assessments, and vigilance toward medical devices associated skin injuries are crucial for patients with injuries like cervical issues. Neglecting them can lead to complications such as skin sores. Effective supervision, regular communication among nursing staff, and adherence to hospital policies are essential to prevent such oversights. Nurses should ensure that appropriate care measures are consistently followed; they must be observant toward the possibility of medical devices associated skin injuries, and should promptly address any issues or concerns related to patient care during shift handovers.

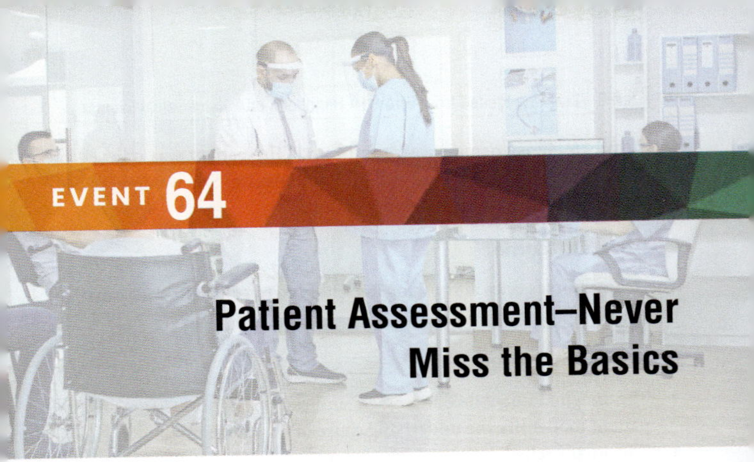

EVENT 64

Patient Assessment–Never Miss the Basics

EVENT NO.	PSE/064/092022
IPSG RELATED TO	None

CASE STUDY DESCRIPTION

A 62-year-old lady underwent total knee replacement, and the surgery was successful. On the 4th postoperative day, the patient complained of discomfort, loose motion, loss of appetite, and refused to get herself ambulated. While on rounds, the nursing supervisor, on being told about the patient's complaints, asked the assigned nurse what her interventions were for the patient. The assigned nurse answered that she had informed the resident doctor, and he had prescribed antidiarrheal drugs. However, the senior nurse was not convinced with the intervention and believed there was something more that had not been addressed. Hence, she went back to the patient and asked a few more questions.

When did she last have her bowel movements? The patient replied that it was two days ago.

Was she comfortable after her bowel movements? The patient answered that she feels she has not emptied her bowel even after the bowel movement. Frequently she was passing a small amount of watery stool.

The senior nurse identified that the patient had impacted stool and the loose motion was the liquid part seeping around the impacted stool.

The patient was counselled that she required a rectal examination. The doctor did the rectal exam and removed the impacted stool. Following this, a proctoclysis enema was administered. The patient was relieved of her distress and started eating well and ambulating. She was prescribed laxatives and advised to drink plenty of liquids.

Positive Outcome

The senior nurse's critical thinking and probing to get to the root cause of the patient's problem.

Errors Encountered

- The assigned nurse failed to assess and ask the right questions to the patient to identify the underlying cause of the problem.
- The doctor relied entirely on the nurse.
- Essential history collection and physical assessments were missed.
- The assigned nurse failed to reassess the patient after the administration of the treatment.

Lessons Learned

For nurse	For nurse educator	For nurse administrator
• Proper history collection and physical examination. Take help from seniors on the areas of doubt. • Focus on assessment and reassessment.	• Train nurses on history collection and also about asking patients the right questions which are essential to identify patients' problems correctly. • Teach techniques of physical examination. • Such incidents can be used as training topics.	The department can institute recognition program where assigned nurses exhibits critical thinking and takes proactive measures in the interest of the patient.

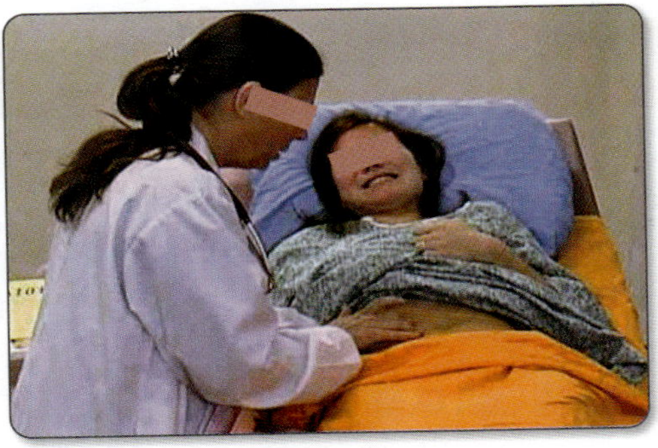

Figure 64 Abdominal examination

Event-Based Learning Summary

This case serves as a reminder of the importance of thorough patient assessments and critical thinking in nursing care. Nurses should never overlook the basics, such as detailed history collection, physical examination, and the use of essential medical instruments like a stethoscope. In this instance, a senior nurse's critical thinking and in-depth assessment uncovered the root cause of the patient's discomfort, demonstrating the significance of continuous vigilance. It emphasizes that nurses should not rely solely on prescribed medications but should engage in holistic patient care, including identifying and addressing the underlying issues to ensure patient well-being. Furthermore, reassessment after interventions is crucial to monitor the effectiveness of the treatment.

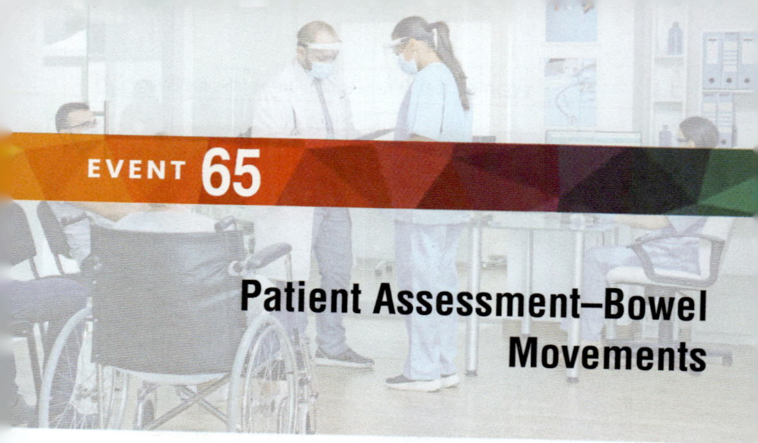

EVENT 65

Patient Assessment–Bowel Movements

EVENT NO.	PSE/065/092022
IPSG RELATED TO	None

CASE STUDY DESCRIPTION

A 48-year-old male patient was admitted after a fall from bike with pain, swelling, and bruising over the left leg. Radiological and clinical features suggested fracture tibia and soft tissue injury. He was posted for surgery on the day of his admission. However his surgery was postponed 3 times and the patient had received suppositories for cleansing his bowel for all three days. On the fourth day, the patient underwent open reduction and internal fixation (ORIF). First postoperative day morning, he was prescribed a suppository again by the physician. The assigned nurse delegated the task to a junior nurse. The patient refused to have it administered. The nurse informed the senior nurse and withheld the treatment.

Positive Outcome

None.

Errors Encountered

- Patient was not asked clearly about his bowel and bladder movements during the morning rounds.

- The assigned nurse did not have a complete picture of the patient's stay in the hospital. Hence, she could not remind the doctor that he had been getting suppositories for three consecutive days.
- Incomplete nursing assessment.

Lessons Learned

For nurse	For nurse educator	For nurse administrator
• Assigned nurses must know the complete history of the patient and one of the basic question the nurse should ask to the patient is about the elimination. • It is important the nurse must enquire about patient's last bowel movement and frequency when nurses are asked to administer laxatives. • When nurses are aware of complete history they can prevent any oversight from the doctors. • Focus on assessment and reassessment.	• During training emphasize to nurses on importance of asking basic questions about patient's intake and elimination, whenever they take handover of patients. • Teach techniques of physical examination.	The nurse administrator should not forget to share learnings from such incidents with other nurses in the department.

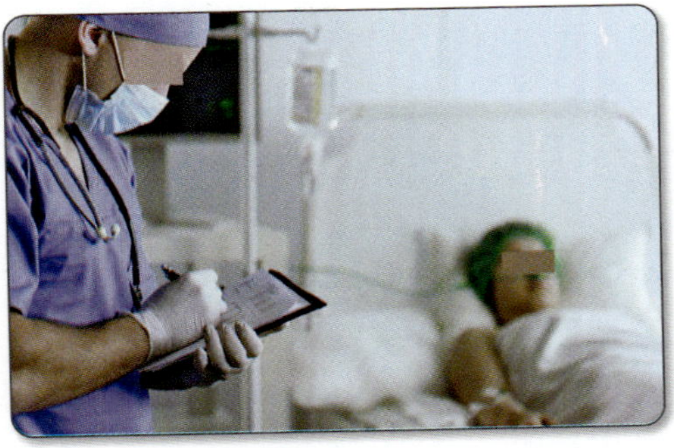

Figure 65 Assessment of patient postoperatively

Event-Based Learning Summary

This case underscores the importance of effective communication and comprehensive patient assessment in nursing care. Nurses should always ask patients about their experiences and medical history, taking into consideration any procedures or medications they have received in the past. In this scenario, a junior nurse's attentive approach and willingness to clarify the patient's needs led to the patient's refusal of a suppository that he no longer required. Furthermore, another nurse's inquiry regarding the patient's previous treatment history helped prevent an unnecessary procedure, highlighting the significance of open communication among the healthcare team. Ultimately, nurses should always strive to obtain a complete and up-to-date patient history to provide the best possible care.

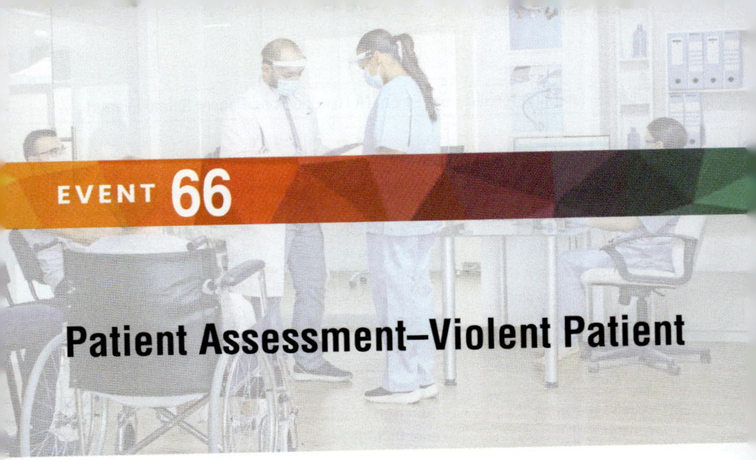

EVENT 66

Patient Assessment–Violent Patient

EVENT NO.	PSE/066/092022
IPSG RELATED TO	None

CASE STUDY DESCRIPTION

A 30-year-old female patient was admitted to a psychiatric department in a private ward with Paranoid Schizophrenia who was aggressive and violent by nature. One day the TV in her room was not working, and the patient started yelling at everyone using abusive words. She came to the nurse's station and shouted at the nurses. At that moment, a new trainee nurse was on her first day at work and found the situation amusing and started laughing. This made the patient even angrier. She insulted and tried to attack the nurse.

Positive Outcome

Senior nurses understood the patient's disease condition, respected the patient because of her illness, and stayed calm.

Error Encountered

The trainee nurse laughed at the patient's behavior thereby making the patient more angry.

Lessons Learned

For nurse	For nurse educator	For nurse administrator
• When we encounter a violent and aggressive patient, we should stay calm, firm, and composed. • Ensure personal safety. • Call for help. • Assess the patient for signs of distress or potential triggers for their behavior. • Use de-escalation techniques: Such as active listening, empathy, and offering choices. • Follow facility policy.	• Any nurse when assigned to a psychiatric ward must have a special orientation before deploying them for handling mentally ill patients. • Induction program must include lessons on the role of nurses in psychiatry ward, communication skills, patient management, crisis intervention techniques, etc. • Provide hands-on training.	• SOPs to be defined on handling agitated patient and skill distribution also to be looked at. Acuity based patient allocation to be done. • Ensure new nurses are provided with clear job descriptions and requirements when assigned to the psychiatric patients. • Provide ongoing support and mentorship.

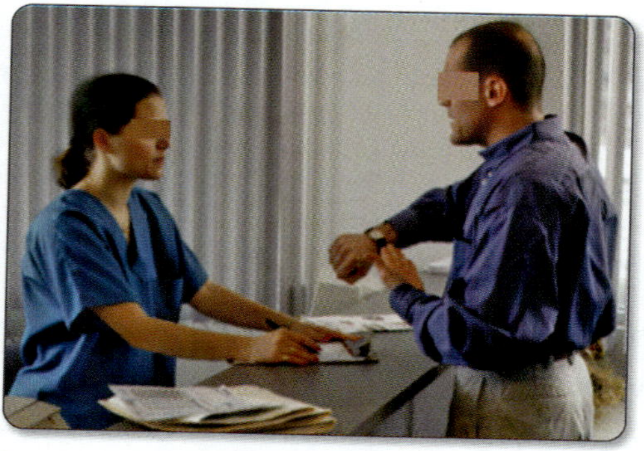

Figure 66 Nurse should be calm when handling aggressive patient

Event-Based Learning Summary

When dealing with psychiatric patients, especially for new trainee nurses, it is essential to provide comprehensive orientation that emphasizes safe behavior and includes a thorough understanding of potential trigger behavior that could agitate the patients. In this case, the trainee nurse's inappropriate reaction, laughter, escalated the patient's aggression. Senior nurses who understood the patient's condition remained calm and handled the situation appropriately. Respect, empathy, and proper training are vital when working with individuals suffering from mental illnesses to ensure their safety and well-being, as well as that of the healthcare team.

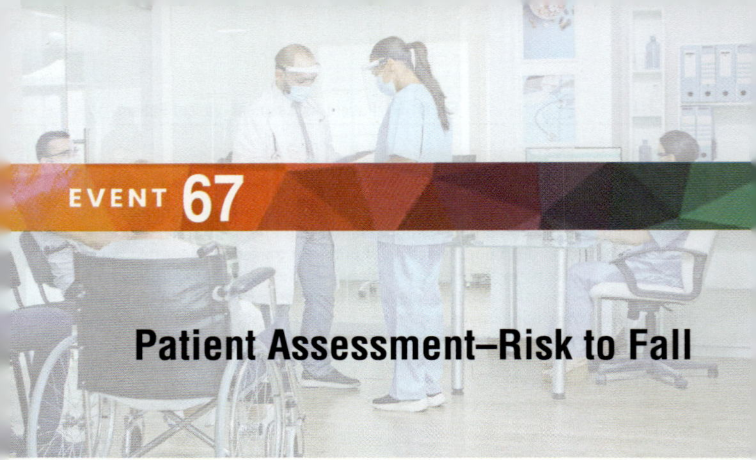

EVENT 67

Patient Assessment–Risk to Fall

EVENT NO.	PSE/067/092022
IPSG RELATED TO	None

CASE STUDY DESCRIPTION

An 80-year-old male brought to the emergency room after a fall at home. He had a history of severe dementia and osteoporosis. The patient was admitted to the bed which was 20 feet away from nursing station. A registered nurse assessed the patient and documented that the patient was confused, uncooperative and identified the risk of falls. Two hours later the patient had given sedatives for a diagnostic test to assess head, knees, pelvis and ribs, the results were negative. 30 minutes later the patient was found lying on the floor to the right side of the bed. The patient underwent additional diagnostic tests, confirmed a fractured right hip. The patient underwent an open reduction and internal fixation of his hip fracture. The patient was able to ambulate prior to this hospitalization, but his activity level is now limited to a wheelchair.

Positive Outcome

None.

Errors Encountered

Failure to employ fall prevention measures. Despite the patient being at high-risk for fall.

Lessons Learned

For nurse	For nurse educator	For nurse administrator
• Have periodic monitoring and insist an attender to stay back with patient at all times. • Request senior to keep such high-risk patients closer to the nursing station.	• Train nurses on fall prevention measures. • Demonstrate fall prevention techniques, such as assessing the patient's fall risk, using appropriate equipment, and creating a safe environment. • Use case studies: Case studies can help trainees to understand the complex factors that can contribute to falls and develop effective strategies for preventing falls. • Engage in role-playing exercises: Role-playing exercises can help trainees to practice implementing fall prevention techniques in a simulated environment.	• Develop a comprehensive fall prevention program that includes assessment tools, policies and procedures, and staff education and training. • Use technology such as alarms and sensors. • Collaborate with interdisciplinary teams. • Involve patients and families in the fall prevention program by providing education. • Monitor and track falls using a standardized reporting system to identify patterns and trends.

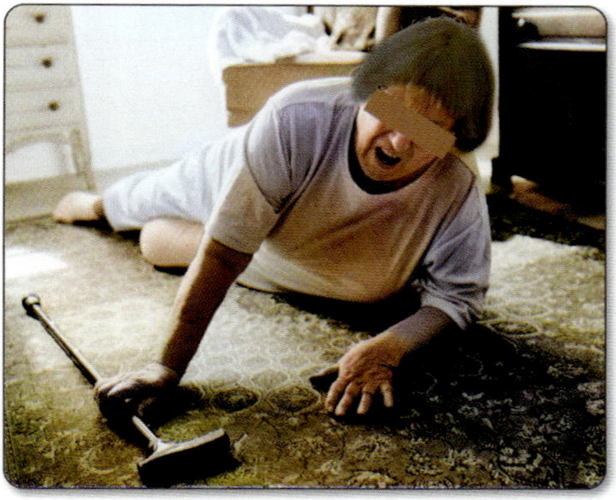

Figure 67 Teach the patient and family member about fall prevention strategies

Event-Based Learning Summary

In the case of an elderly patient with severe dementia and osteoporosis, risk assessment for falls is crucial. While the initial nursing assessment identified the risk for falls, a subsequent lapse in monitoring allowed the patient to fall, resulting in a fractured right hip. It is essential to consistently and attentively monitor patients at risk of falling, especially when they have additional complications. Prompt interventions and strict adherence to protocols can help prevent such accidents and their associated consequences.

Furthermore, in cases involving patients at high risk of falls, especially those with conditions like severe dementia and osteoporosis, actively engaging both the patient and their family in fall prevention measures is crucial. Nurses should ensure that the patient's family is educated about the elevated risk of falls and the potential serious harm that can result. Family involvement, education, and awareness play a pivotal role in reinforcing preventive measures and maintaining patient safety during their hospital stay.

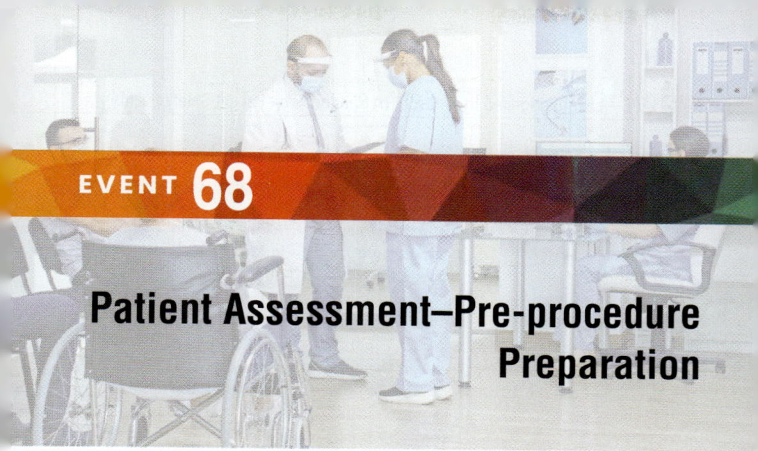

EVENT 68

Patient Assessment–Pre-procedure Preparation

EVENT NO.	PSE/068/092022
IPSG RELATED TO	None

CASE STUDY DESCRIPTION

A 39-year-old female admitted with complaints of abdominal pain, nausea, and mild abdominal distention from past 6 months. She had history of consumption of alcohol and tobacco. She was diagnosed with cardiomegaly, pericholecystic fluid, moderate pleural effusion and early pancreatitis. The gastroenterologist scheduled a EUS/ERCP after cardiac evaluation but the procedure was done without the cardiac evaluation. During the procedure, the patient collapsed and despite of all resuscitative measures patient could not be saved.

An autopsy was performed, and the report indicated that the patient died due to severe cardiomyopathy and moderate pulmonary edema.

Positive Outcome

None.

Errors Encountered

- Failure to carry out the preoperative order.
- Negligence of healthcare provider in counter checking the orders.
- Failure of the healthcare team to do follow-up.

Lessons Learned

For nurse	For nurse educator	For nurse administrator
• Ensure preoperative orders are carried out and verified • Identify the risk factors and escalate to all stakeholders.	• Ensure nurses are trained on pre-procedural orders that can be unique for certain diagnosis. • Use such events to highlight the need for nurses to be diligent to ensure all pre-op work up is completed before shifting patient for the procedure.	Taking cue from this unfortunate event nurse leader can plan to introduce the pre-procedural checklist (similar to pre-op checklist). This checklist can ensure the team carries out all the pre-procedural orders.

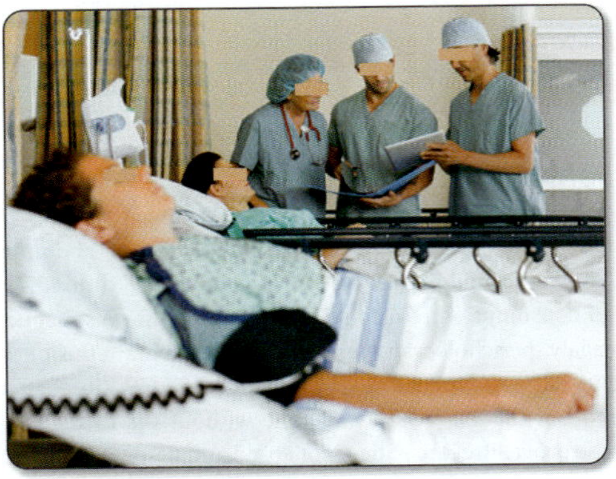

Figure 68 Nurses ensuring preoperative orders are verified prior to surgery

Event-Based Learning Summary

This case underscores the importance of adhering to preprocedure orders, meticulous documentation, effective communication, and patient advocacy in nursing practice. Neglecting essential preprocedure assessments and failing to follow-up on orders can have serious consequences. Nurses must prioritize patient safety by ensuring all necessary evaluations are completed, advocating for their patients and maintaining clear records. Additionally, a culture of continuous learning and quality improvement is vital to prevent similar incidents in the future.

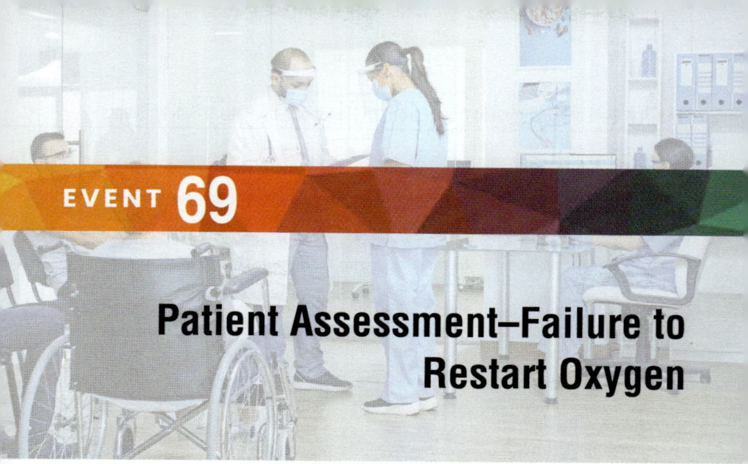

EVENT 69

Patient Assessment–Failure to Restart Oxygen

EVENT NO.	PSE/069/092022
IPSG RELATED TO	None

CASE STUDY DESCRIPTION

Baby Aysha, 4 years/F, was admitted to the pediatric ward with bronchial asthma. She was on oxygen 2 L/min *via* nasal prongs. She was afebrile, pulse 98 beats/min, respiratory rate 36/min. Since she had to have food, the oxygen administration was stopped for a few minutes; and the nasal prongs were kept aside. After having food, the staff forgot to reconnect the nasal prongs.

Meanwhile, another nurse went and reconnected the nasal prongs. After an hour, when the pediatrician came for rounds, he noted that the oxygen was not flowing.

Positive Outcomes

- The pediatrician found that the oxygen was not flowing, and it was restarted without delay.
- The patient did not suffer with any serious complications.

Errors Encountered

The nurse did not open the valve of the oxygen cylinder after reconnecting the nasal prongs.

Lessons Learned

For nurse	For nurse educator	For nurse administrator
• To remain attentive and vigilant while doing procedure. • To verify on the functioning of apparatus. • Involve patient attendant with the children and educate them on treatment and interventions being done for their child. This will ensure the attendant reminds of any delay in restarting the oxygen.	Use such events to sensitize nurse to be diligent throughout the duty hours.	Ensure that such events are discussed in all nursing groups to sensitize nurses on potential harm that can be done if the nurses are not diligent around patients.

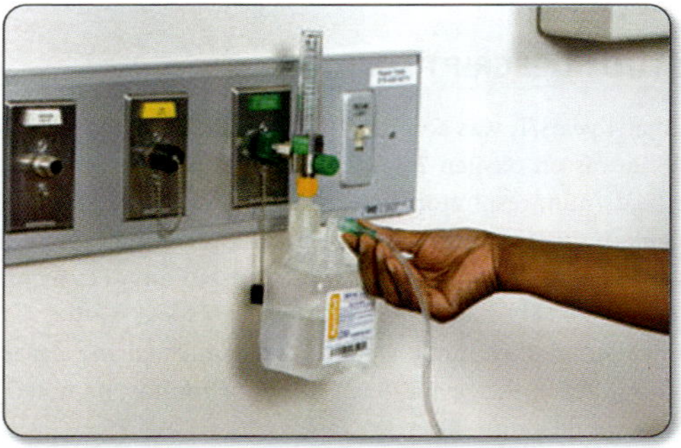

Figure 69 Nurse ensures the functioning of oxygen humidifier

Event-Based Learning Summary

In this case, the nurse's oversight in reconnecting oxygen to a pediatric patient with bronchial asthma highlights the critical need for vigilant monitoring. Thankfully, the pediatrician detected the error promptly, preventing potential severe complications. This incident underscores the importance of timely recognition and correction of patient care lapses to ensure patient safety. Nurses must remain diligent and attentive to all aspects of care, especially when dealing with vulnerable pediatric patients.

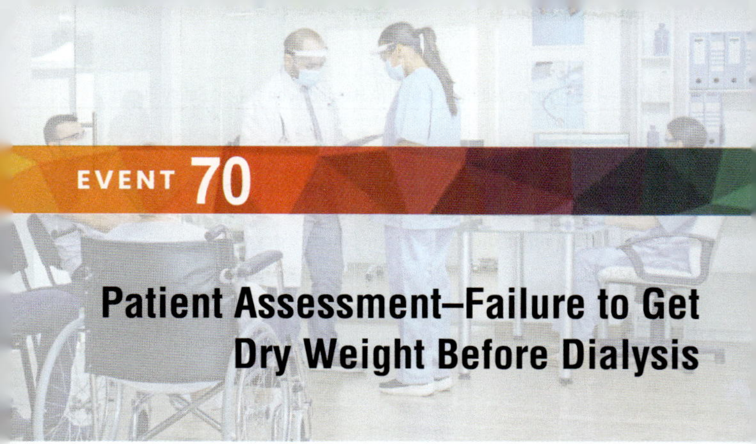

EVENT 70

Patient Assessment–Failure to Get Dry Weight Before Dialysis

EVENT NO.	PSE/070/092022
IPSG RELATED TO	None

CASE STUDY DESCRIPTION

Mr Saravanan, a 50-year-old male patient with chronic kidney disease (CKD) was on regular dialysis. One day the patient came to the dialysis unit with the complaints of severe dyspnea. The assigned nurse immediately shifted the patient to the dialysis chair and started the dialysis process with the regular fluid removal volume UF goal-1000 mL She neither consulted with unit doctor neither done the patient assessment. After the dialysis session, the patient was sent back home. After 6 hours the patient had developed mild dyspnea again. The patient returned to hospital from home and consulted the doctors for his complaints. After the reassessment, the doctor advised to remove an additional 500 mL fluid. The doctor identified that the assigned nurse didn't assess the patient's dry weight. After the second session of dialysis, the patient's condition got stabilized and discharged.

Positive Outcome

Reassessment was done and removed additional 500 mL of fluid.

Errors Encountered

- The assigned nurse started dialysis without doing a patient assessment.
- The nurse didn't consult the unit doctor.
- The assigned nurse didn't assess the patient's dry weight.

Lessons Learned

For nurse	For nurse educator	For nurse administrator
• The nurses should never deviate from established protocol specially with the patients who are on dialysis. • Educate patient and family the importance of taking weight before dialysis.	• Training on importance of pre and post procedure assessment. • During training emphasize on patient assessment and re-assessment.	Structured documentation to summarize the entire dialysis event starting from pre, intra and post procedure event and assessments.

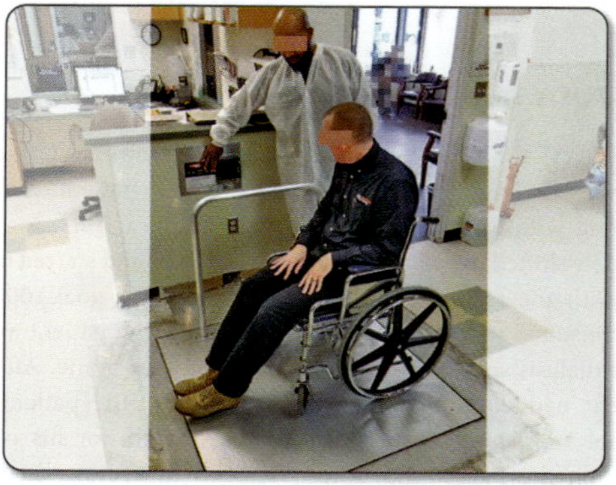

Figure 70 Checking dry weight of patient before dialysis

Event-Based Learning Summary

This incident underscores the critical importance of proper patient assessment and communication in a dialysis unit. The assigned nurse initiated a dialysis procedure without assessing the patient and failed to consult the unit doctor, leading to complications. Failure to determine the patient's dry weight resulted in postdialysis dyspnea, emphasizing the need for diligent predialysis assessments and communication with the healthcare team to ensure safe and effective patient care during dialysis. Such incidents stress the significance of thorough patient evaluation before initiating medical procedures.

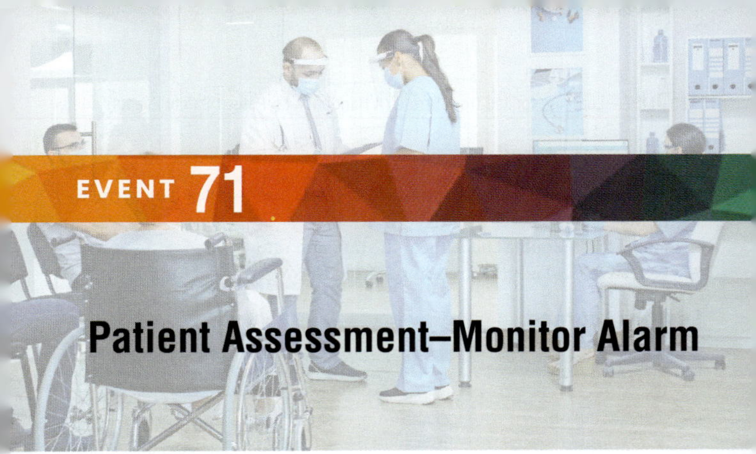

EVENT 71

Patient Assessment–Monitor Alarm

EVENT NO.	PSE/071/092022
IPSG RELATED TO	None

CASE STUDY DESCRIPTION

A 3-year-old child underwent neurosurgery and was shifted to ICU for observation. The child was electively intubated and sedated. The ICU was a mixed one admitting mostly adults and occasionally pediatric patients. The pediatric surgeon ordered 20 mL of fluids to be infused per hour. The assigned nurse connected the child to monitor, and the volumetric pump was used to infuse the fluid. After half an hour, the nurse noticed sudden tachycardia in the child's vital parameters and immediately notified the unit in-charge. Both started their immediate assessment. Since the child was sedated, it was challenging to assess the child's level of consciousness; however, on chest auscultation, they identified crepitus. The lungs were filled with fluid, and on checking the IV pump, they realised that the fluid was being delivered at 200 mL/hr instead of 20 mL. The ICU intensivist was notified immediately, and the child was administered Inj. Lasix, which saved the child.

Positive Outcomes

- The assigned nurse was quick and alert to identify the immediate changes in heart rate and notified her senior without any delay.
- Critical thinking and quick assessment helped to determine the cause of the problem.

Errors Encountered

- The Volumetric infusion pump (VIP) was used instead of syringe pump.
- Failed to do double checking of the infusion rate.
- Excessive fluid administration resulting in congestion of lungs.

Lessons Learned

For nurse	For nurse educator	For nurse administrator
• When smaller volumes are ordered always use syringe pump. • Insist senior nurses/in-charge to cross verify. • When assigned to unfamiliar category of patients always get a senior to double check every intervention.	• While training ICU nurses, nurses must be warned that they are trained to look after the specific category of patients. • Hence, if at any time they are required to look after another category of patients nurses must seek supervision and get every action double checked.	• Plan for age-specific and specialty specific ICUs to prevent such error. • When in emergency if nurses have to look after other category of patient, senior nurses must be directed to provide supervision and guidance. • Competency and privileging of nurses must be known and respected by the senior nurses. • In case there is no option except mixed ICU, the nurses must be specially trained for age-specific competencies.

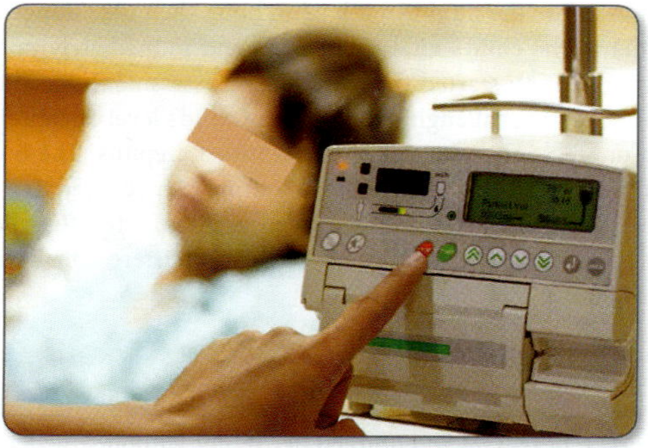

Figure 71 Handling of pediatric cases on fluid therapy through infusion pump

Event-Based Learning Summary

This case emphasizes the crucial role of vigilance and double-checking in pediatric care within mixed intensive care units. The nurse's quick identification of abnormal vital signs, collaboration with a senior nurse, and effective assessment skills were pivotal in identifying and resolving the issue of fluid delivery error. However, the incident highlights the need for dedicated pediatric units and specialized training for nurses to ensure focused care and minimize potential errors in an environment where both adults and children are treated. Vigilance and thorough checks in pediatric care are essential to maintain patient safety in mixed ICU settings.

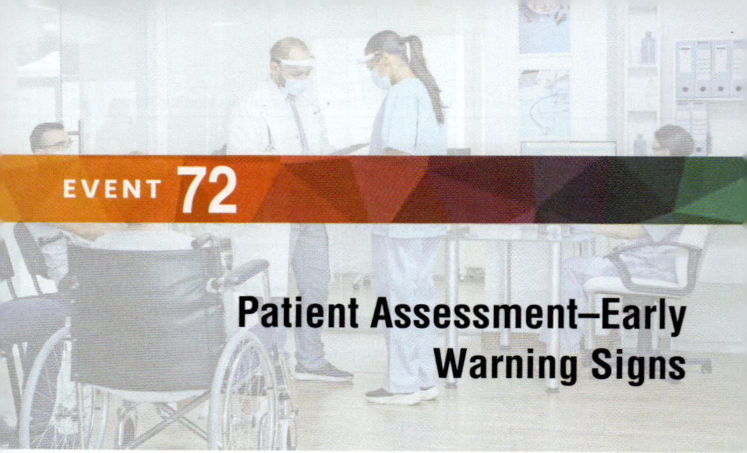

EVENT 72

Patient Assessment–Early Warning Signs

EVENT NO.	PSE/072/092022
IPSG RELATED TO	None

CASE STUDY DESCRIPTION

A 20-day-old twin baby who was 26-week preterm was being cared for in a warmer in Level III Nursery. The baby was diagnosed with cerebral edema with bilateral grade 4 severe Intra Ventricular Hemorrhage and Central Diabetes Insipidus with a heart rate of 124/min, respiratory rate 44/min, saturation 98% on room air, appearing pink and hypotonic. The baby was cared for from day 2 of life with the full support of an incubator and ventilator. The baby was on the 37th day of life with 16 mL hourly feeding and Levipil 30 mg/kg/day. The baby was found to have a reddish color change over the skin on the right ear and the scalp in the occipital region. The medical and nursing team were alerted, and Allevyn patch was applied in the occipital region with periodic position changes and emollients to the skin.

Positive Outcome

Consistent care helped in identifying the problem at the earliest.

Errors Encountered

The baby developed pressure injury.

Lessons Learned

For nurse	For nurse educator	For nurse administrator
• When high-risk babies are assigned to the nurses, take proactive measures to prevent even minor changes in the skin. (Allevyn patch could have been applied earlier even before the redness has appeared). • Always seek help/guidance from experienced seniors when caring for such high-risk babies.	When training and privileging nurses for specific ICUs, potential nursing related complications must be included. Use case studies like this to emphasize the need for nurse to be extra vigilant in such high risk units.	• Ensure at least once in every shift the babies are fully assessed by a senior nurse. • Have a process for complete recording and reporting of adverse events while doing RCA.

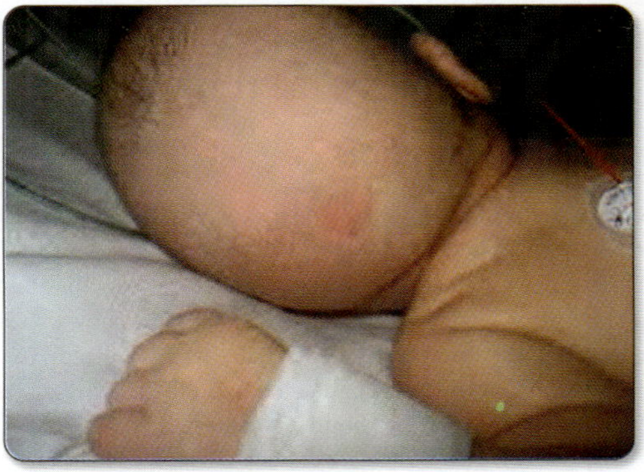

Figure 72 NICU baby positioning is changed every two hourly

Event-Based Learning Summary

In the case of the 20-day-old premature twin baby, early identification and intervention in response to skin changes played a crucial role in preventing a pressure sore. The consistent care and alertness of the medical and nursing teams were key factors in maintaining the baby's skin health and supporting their overall well-being. This case underscores the importance of promoting protective practices and skin care protocols, especially in neonatal care. Taking proactive preventive measure by anticipating that the baby can develop pressure related skin changes could have prevented even before the appearance of redness on the pressure points.

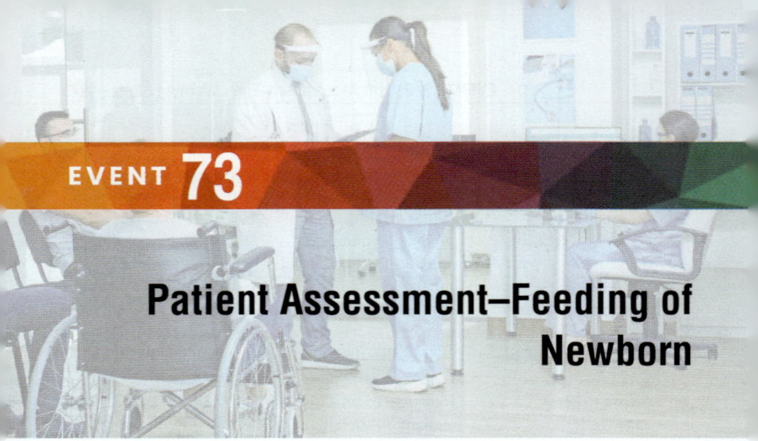

EVENT 73

Patient Assessment–Feeding of Newborn

EVENT NO.	PSE/073/092022
IPSG RELATED TO	None

CASE STUDY DESCRIPTION

A 2-day-old preterm baby of low-birth weight was admitted with the mother. Mother had history of GDM. Early morning at 4:30 am baby was found to have relaxed posture and lethargy. The duty doctor and the floor nursing supervisor were immediately informed and baby was shifted to a warmer unit and started on IV fluid. Baby was stabilized. The nursing supervisor found that the nurse had failed to do the feeding assessment as per the institution's policy (2nd hourly) for the baby.

Positive Outcome

The nurse identified the baby's changing status on time.

Errors Encountered

- Assigned nurse failed to do the feeding assessment 2 hourly.
- The baby went into hypoglycemia and dehydration.

Lessons Learned

For nurse	For nurse educator	For nurse administrator
• When assigned to neonates the nurses need to ensure the baby is fed at regular interval as per departmental policy. • Be aware that these very young patients have little reserve for food and fluid.	• Train nurse on feeding assessment 2nd hourly and the rational for the same. • Conduct specialized department specific training sessions.	• Assessment chart can be customized indicating the time for assessment. • Periodic audit and review by In charge for the adherence. • Privileged nurses to be assigned for high-risk category of patients.

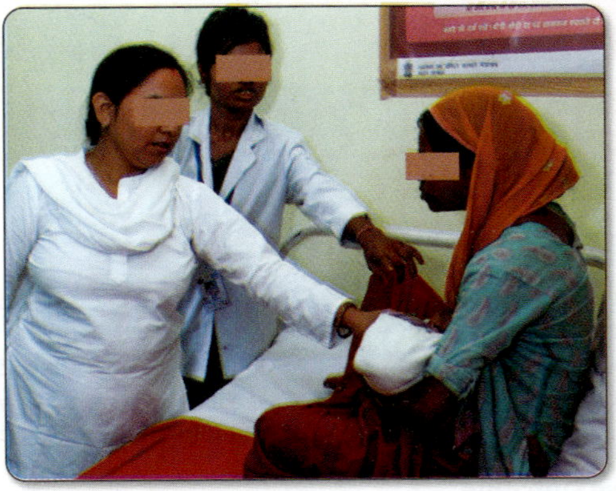

Figure 73 Nurse assessing and teaching mother on breastfeeding

Event-Based Learning Summary

In the case of the 2-day-old term baby boy, the immediate response by the nursing supervisor to address the baby's lethargy and initiate appropriate care, including warmer and IV fluid, was a positive step. However, the assigned nurses failure to follow the feeding assessment policy and conduct regular assessments, along with not educating the mother about feeding, were significant shortcomings. Effective and timely assessments and patient education are crucial in neonatal care to ensure the well-being of both the newborn and the mother.

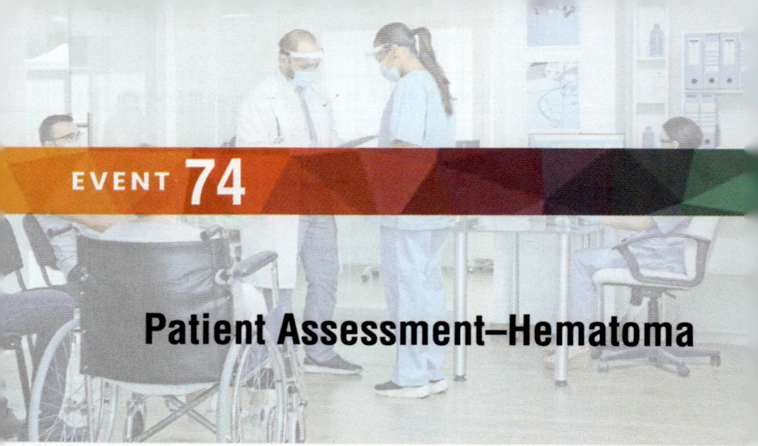

EVENT 74

Patient Assessment–Hematoma

EVENT NO.	PSE/074/092022
IPSG RELATED TO	None

CASE STUDY DESCRIPTION

A 36-year-old patient was admitted with complaints of fever and chills. The patient's platelet count was 73 thousand and her PT INR was 0.9. She developed hematoma in the antecubital fossa after a blood sample collection by a laboratory technician. Cold compression with ice was given to the affected site, and $MgSO_4$ dressing was done.

Positive Outcome

Hematoma was identified and necessary interventions were initiated.

Errors Encountered

- The laboratory technician did not collect the patient's history and check the last blood results value before the venipuncture procedure.
- The assigned nurse did not brief the laboratory technician on the value of the platelets and the risk of patient bleeding.
- The assigned nurse failed to take necessary action to prevent hematoma.

Lessons Learned

For nurse	For nurse educator	For nurse administrator
• The assigned nurse must be aware of the risk associated with patients diagnosis and abnormal test values. • These information must be used by the assigned nurse to collaborate with the healthcare workers to prevent patient harm. • The nurse could have warned the lab technician and assisted in ensuring adequate pressure to prevent bleeding and hematoma. • Monitor the site. • Educate patient and attendant on the potential risk and report any changes without delay.	• Training nurses on vein puncture and sample collection procedures must highlight high-risk patients where extra vigilance and monitoring is required. • Demonstrate how to apply pressure dressing to prevent bleeding and hematoma. • Remind nurses to take charge of their patient by providing timely warning and assistance to other healthcare team members who would be involved in their patient care.	Alert board or band can be incorporated to communicate patient risks within the healthcare team members.

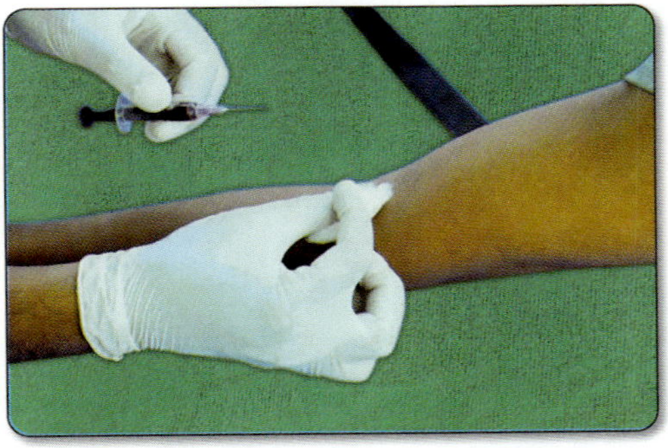

Figure 74 Applying pressure after collection of blood sample to prevent hematoma

Event-Based Learning Summary

Nurses are pivotal in ensuring patient safety, and one proactive step which they can take is to inform phlebotomists about potential risk factors, such as low platelet counts, before blood collection procedures. Nurses, as constant patient caregivers, should act as advocates and champions for patient safety, fostering effective communication within the healthcare team. By being vigilant about patients' medical histories and conditions, nurses can identify and address potential risks, ultimately enhancing patient safety and care quality. This collaborative approach among healthcare providers prioritizes patient well-being, making it essential in healthcare delivery.

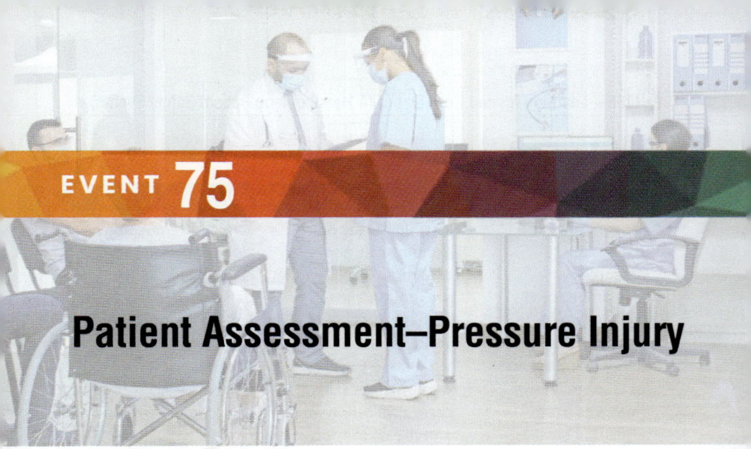

EVENT 75

Patient Assessment–Pressure Injury

EVENT NO.	PSE/075/092022
IPSG RELATED TO	None

CASE STUDY DESCRIPTION

A 68-year-old, semiconscious, bedridden, thinly built patient was admitted to CCU on July 20, 2021 with endocarditis, severe Left Ventricular dysfunction, stage V CKD on Hemodialysis and severe diarrhea. He was noticed to have developed a **Grade I Pressure** injury on 22nd July.

Positive Outcome

None.

Error Encountered

The assigned nurses failed to identify the high-risk factors of the patient to develop pressure injury. Hence failed to adopt preventive measures on time.

Lessons Learned

For nurse	For nurse educator	For nurse administrator
• Perform physical assessment including skin assessment of all pressure points in every shift for all vulnerable patients. • Initiate preventive measures from admission such as – 2-hrly repositioning, pressure relieving mattress, preventing pressure friction, shear and moisture.	• To train nurses on Braden scale and pressure ulcer prevention and management. • Train on care of vulnerable patients. • Demonstrate skin care, application and use of comfort devices for at-risk patients. • Use case studies and scenarios to teach.	• To institute position clock and monitoring for the bed-ridden patients. • Ensure the documented handover during the shift change. • Ensure frequent rounds are conducted by the nurse supervisor and the in-charge. • Safety rounds conducted by the seniors must include physical assessment of high-risk patients and implementation of the correct nursing care plan. • Communicate with the patient and their companions. • Review incidents and analyse the most common causes. • Acuity-based assignment of patient.

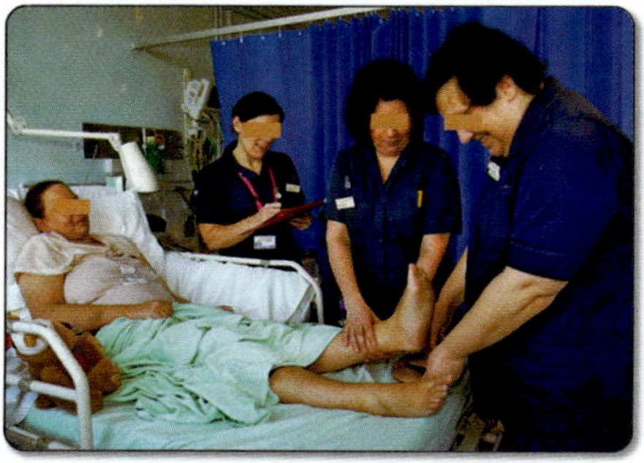

Figure 75 Nursing team assessing risk of pressure ulcer

Event-Based Learning Summary

This incident emphasizes the importance of training all nurses about the heightened risk critically ill patients face in developing pressure injuries. Shift-charged nurses should provide guidance and supervision to novice nurses. Experienced nurse leaders should have the foresight to anticipate the need for increased supervision and guidance for new nurses rather than placing blame after an adverse event. Regular briefings led by team leaders on patients at risk of complications in the intensive care unit can significantly enhance patient safety and prevent avoidable harm.

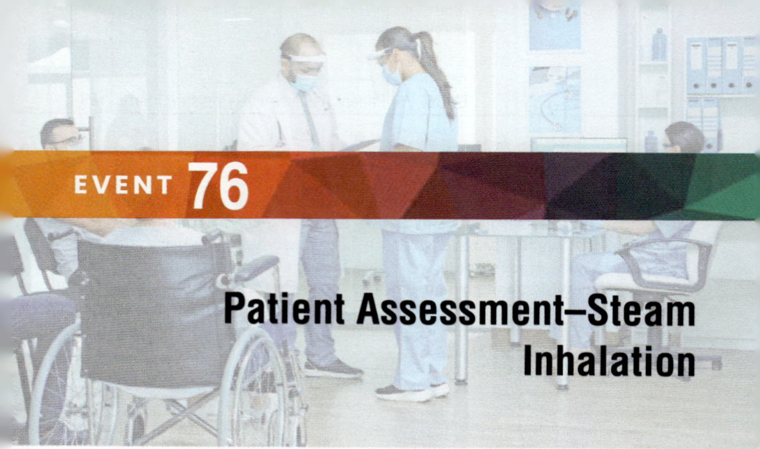

EVENT 76

Patient Assessment–Steam Inhalation

EVENT NO.	PSE/076/092022
IPSG RELATED TO	None

CASE STUDY DESCRIPTION

A 21-year-old male patient was admitted with the diagnosis of CKD. The patient was of very lean and thin built and had lung congestion. The doctor had ordered steam inhalation for his lung congestion.

The nurse prepared for the procedure with all the articles and took Nelson's inhaler to the patient's bedside. Meanwhile, the patient's mother had gone out to buy food. The nurse had kept Nelson's inhaler on the pillow, that was placed on the patient's lap. One of her colleagues called her to enquire about the medication for another patient. She had to leave the patient alone with Nelson's inhaler on his lap. The patient did not hold the Nelson's inhaler properly, and it fell on the patient's legs, which resulted in first-degree burn.

Positive Outcome

None.

Errors Encountered

- She left the patient alone while doing this procedure without realizing the consequences of an adverse event of a burn.
- The patient sustained first degree burn.

Lessons Learned

For nurse	For nurse educator	For nurse administrator
• Assess patient condition before doing any procedure. • Avoid distractions while performing any procedures. • Do not leave the patient alone during a procedure. • The inhaler should be kept on the cardiac table.	Train nurses on preprocedure and postprocedure assessments.	• Have SOPs for all the nursing procedures and postprocedure assessment. • Conduct root cause analysis for such incidents and implement risk mitigating actions. • During training highlight the potential risk of burns.

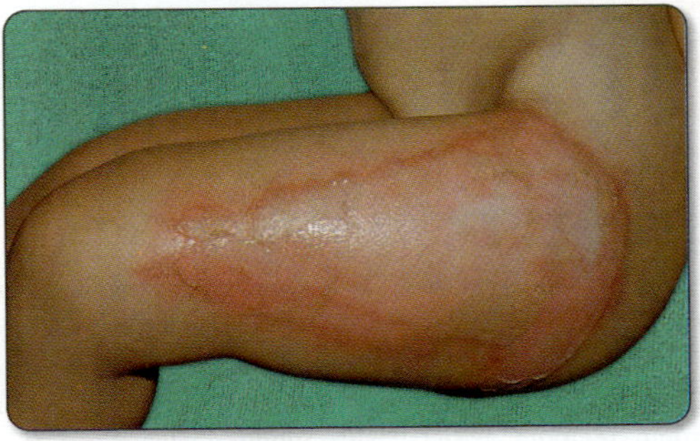

Figure 76 First-degree burn due to fall of Nelson inhaler on legs

Event-Based Learning Summary

This incident underscores the critical importance of patient safety in healthcare. Nurses, especially fresh graduate nurses, must prioritize patient safety above all else. Having situational awareness and realizing that every treatment, even the simplest ones, which are unfamiliar for patients are crucial. Hence, providing thorough patient education before initiating any procedure, warning to patients about potential risks, and emphasizing their role in the process are vital aspects of care. Nurses should maintain constant vigilance, as there is no point in a patient's treatment where they can let their guard down. Patient safety remains paramount throughout their care journey.

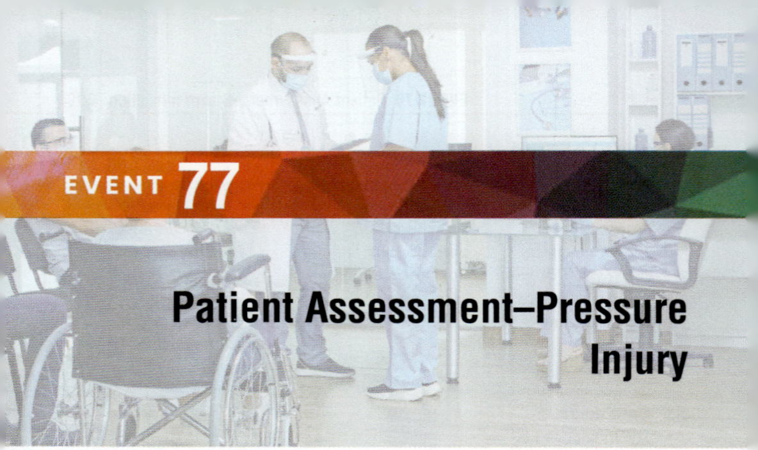

EVENT 77

Patient Assessment–Pressure Injury

EVENT NO.	PSE/077/092022
IPSG RELATED TO	None

CASE STUDY DESCRIPTION

Mr Rangaraj, a 46-year-old male came to emergency medical department with complaints of head injury with bleeding due to road traffic accident (RTA). Immediate assessment was done and necessary treatment was started. The patient was diagnosed with severe traumatic brain injury right Fronto-Temporal parietal with Subdural Hematoma (SDH) and Type 2 DM. On the next day he underwent special procedure of right frontotemporoparietal decompressive craniotomy and tracheostomy was done. Patient had GCS of 9/15 on 39th postoperative day. Patient gradually developed black discoloration of the skin with skin peel in the sacral region. Skin peeling was because of pressure injury.

Positive Outcomes

- The ward in-charge nurse observed during his regular rounds that the patient had developed pressure injury on the sacral region.
- Immediately the charge nurse informed the incident to the treating doctor without any delay to prevent further complication.
- The nursing care plan was revised and care of pressure injury site was started.

Errors Encountered

- Failure to execute Braden scale assessment correctly.
- Failure to anticipate the increased risk of pressure injury due to the medical condition.
- Failure to implement preventive actions.

Lessons Learned

For nurse	For nurse educator	For nurse administrator
• Do Braden scale assessment diligently along with skin assessment of pressure points. • Implement preventive strategies (repositioning, appropriate pressure relieving mattress, care of pressure points, nutrition and hydration) • When patient is restless, additional padding of heel, elbows etc can be useful.	• Train nurses on bed sore assessment scale. • Train all nursing staff on regular inspection of the skin sites for pressure injury.	• Robust SOP on pressure injury assessment, prevention and management. • Ensure availability of the pressure relieving devices at all times. • Conduct regular surprise audits for the vulnerable patients. • Implement process of senior nurses observing pressure points at-least once in a day.

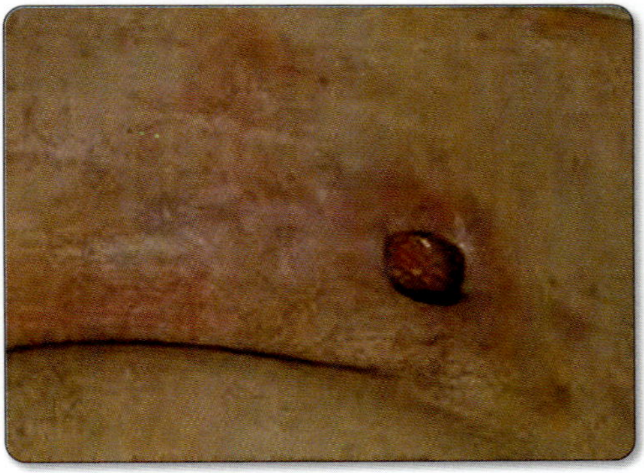

Figure 77 Bedsore at sacrum region

Event-Based Learning Summary

The key takeaways from this case stress the importance of effective communication and collaboration within the healthcare team. While recognizing the doctor's order not to change the patient's position due to postsurgery concerns, nurses should engage in open discussions to assess the risk of pressure injury. These collaborative conversations can lead to the development of innovative preventive measures to avoid pressure injuries in the first place.

Additionally, performing the Braden Scale assessment correctly is utmost important. This assessment provides the foundation for creating an appropriate nursing plan aimed at reducing and mitigating the patient's risk of developing pressure injuries. Healthcare professionals must prioritize accurate assessments and use them as a basis for proactive patient care.

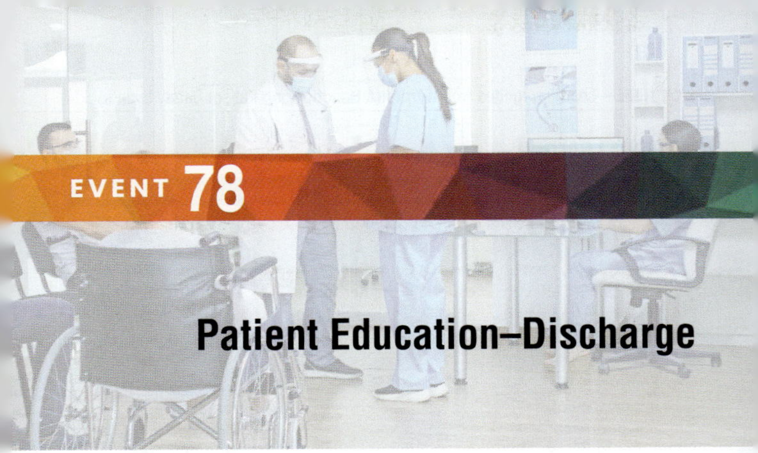

EVENT 78

Patient Education–Discharge

EVENT NO.	PSE/078/092022
IPSG RELATED TO	IPSG 2 – Improve Effective Communication

CASE STUDY DESCRIPTION

A 76-year-old female, a known case of hypertension, was admitted to the ICU. She has been on Tab. Telma 40 mg since 15 years. The patient reported to the hospital complaining of headache, shortness of breath, nasal bleeding, chest pain, and irregular heartbeat. Her blood pressure was noted to be 190/100 mm Hg. In history, it was learned that she did not take her hypertensive medicine at home for >2 weeks.

Positive Outcomes

- The patient is hospitalized, and the correct treatment is started at the right time.
- Antihypertensive medicine was restarted.

Errors Encountered

- The patient had stopped her antihypertensive medicine at home for two weeks.
- Lack of education on critical need for continuing any hypertensive medicine.
- Failed to advise patient not to stop antihypertensive medicine on their own.

Lessons Learned

For nurse	For nurse educator	For nurse administrator
• Ensure the patient is educated on medications, their actions, side effects and when and where to seek help in case of any doubt. • Emphasize the importance of not stopping antihypertensive medications without doctors advise. • Use Teach-Back technique to confirm understanding. • Involve patient's family members/caregivers in this process. • Us teach-back.	Train nurses on the importance of patient specific education especially on medication and importance of using Teach-Back technique.	• Create SOP to deliver clear and complete discharge education. • Emphasize that discharge education should not be kept for the last day, rather it can start from the day of admission. • Condition specific education for patient and attendant handout can be made available in the hospital.

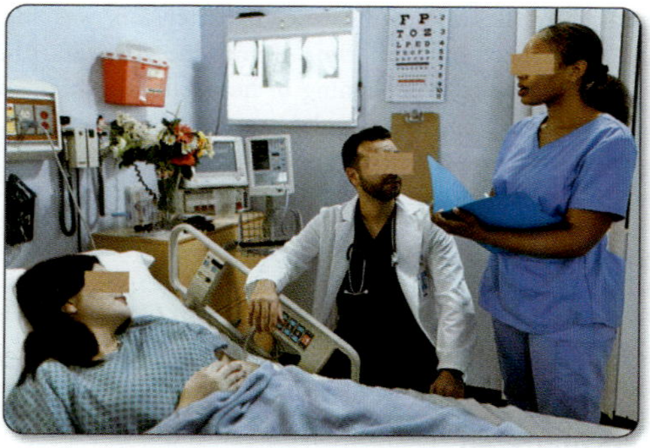

Figure 78 Discharge education given by nurse

Event-Based Learning Summary

This case emphasizes the crucial need for patient education, particularly regarding medication compliance. The patient's failure to take her antihypertensive medication at home for over 2 weeks led to severe health complications. Ensuring that patients understand the importance of taking prescribed medications regularly, even when they feel well, is an essential aspect of healthcare. The Teach-Back method is invaluable in confirming that patients and their families genuinely comprehend the instructions. Additionally, it is essential to initiate education about care and medications early in a patient's hospital stay rather than waiting until the discharge day. This approach prevents information overload and ensures that patients and their families retain critical care instructions even amid the excitement or anxiety surrounding discharge.

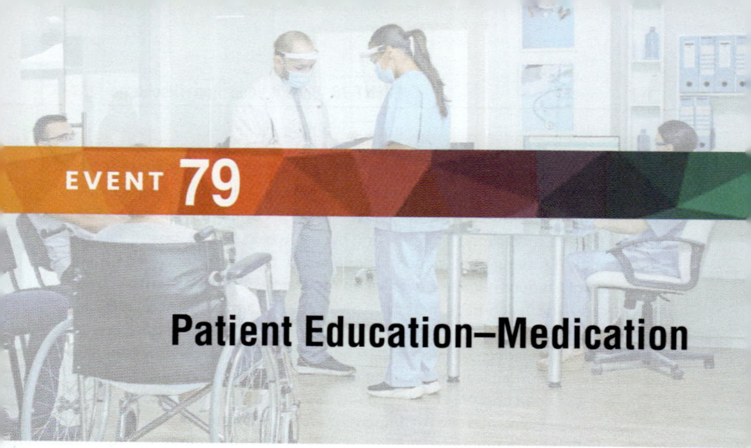

EVENT 79

Patient Education–Medication

EVENT NO.	PSE/079/092022
IPSG RELATED TO	None

CASE STUDY DESCRIPTION

A 63-year-old patient, known case of lung cancer was admitted with severe hyponatremia and disorientation. He was administered 3% NS and was advised to increase his oral salt intake. The doctor advised to fill an empty B Complex capsule shell with salt to ease the consumption of the required additional salt. At the end of four days, the physician noticed that the sodium level had not increased as expected. The physician ordered a costly and highly concentrated medication with sodium. However, the patient's daughter found that the nurse had instructed his family members to empty the B complex capsule's content, mix it with water, and administer it to the patient. The nurse should have explained that the capsule shells need to be refilled with table salt and given to the patient four times a day.*

Positive Outcomes

- The patient was saved from taking a high-dose medication that could have caused various side effects to him.
- The patient's sodium level was finally corrected, and he was fully oriented.

*This practice is an innovative approach suggested by the treating doctor.

Errors Encountered

- The nurse failed to provide the correct explanation to the patient's family.
- The nurse failed to do teach-back and take a written demonstration.
- There is delay in patient recovery.

Lessons Learned

For nurse	For nurse educator	For nurse administrator
• To ensure to educate patients and family on each drug that is being administered. • Ensure the patient and the companions understand the teaching. • Give them the opportunity to repeat back the understanding or redemonstrate the procedure taught • Allow them to ask questions.	Train nurses on the importance of patient specific education and importance of using teach-back and involve family to do return demonstration.	Have a process in place so that nurses can inform any unique method of sodium replacement.

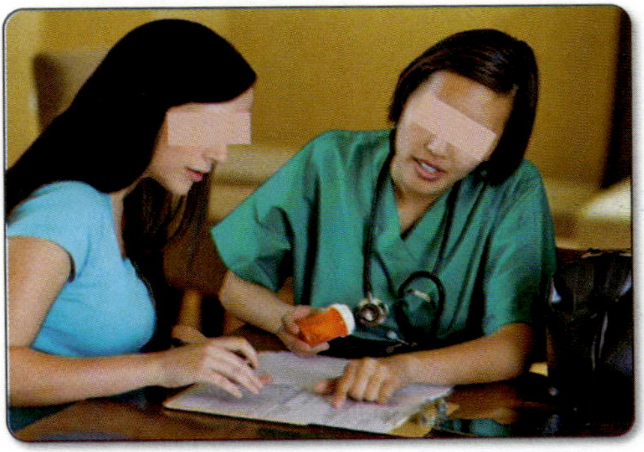

Figure 79 Nurse ensuring patient understands about the teaching

Event-Based Learning Summary

This case underscores the critical role of patient education and communication in ensuring safe and effective healthcare. The nurse's failure to provide accurate and comprehensive instructions to the patient's family regarding the administration of a simple table salt resulted in the doctor's prescribing concentrated saline IV, and this could have resulted in severe side effects. It emphasizes the importance of clear, understandable patient education, coupled with the Teach-Back method, to confirm comprehension. Healthcare providers should anticipate the progress of a patient's condition, ensuring that the prescribed treatment is appropriate and effective. Timely and accurate patient education is paramount in preventing medication errors and enhancing patient safety. Demonstrating any procedure without return demonstration can lead to miscommunication. Additionally, healthcare providers should never assume that patients and families fully understand routine procedures, underlining the need for clear, repeated instruction to ensure patient safety. Asking for a return demonstration in this case would have prevented this error completely.

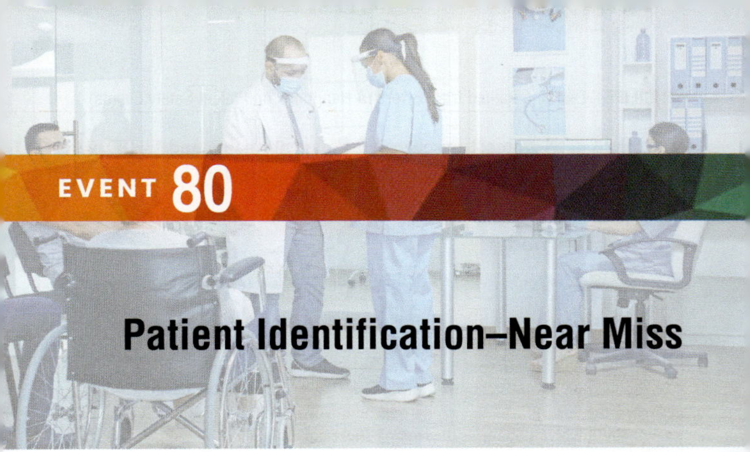

EVENT 80

Patient Identification–Near Miss

EVENT NO.	PSE/080/092022
IPSG RELATED TO	IPSG 1 – Identify the Patient Correctly

CASE STUDY DESCRIPTION

Mrs Reena was diagnosed with postmyocardial infarction, Mrs Revathy was diagnosed with a stroke, and both the patients were admitted to the second floor. Both patients were admitted for further observation and monitoring. Both the patients stayed in the same twin-sharing room. The nurse who was assigned to the room interchanged their medications. Since the patient's attendant was aware of the medicines, the error was noticed immediately and corrected.

Positive Outcomes

- Attender of patient Mrs Reena was well aware of the prescription and rechecked the drugs with the supervisor/in-charge.
- The in-charge nurse has taken immediate action to rectify the problem.
- The right medication was administered to the right patient.

Errors Encountered

- The assigned nurse was not following the 'Rights of Medication Administration'.

- Drug safety protocol on checking a patient's name and UHID with that of medication administration record was not done before the drug administration.

Lessons Learned

For nurse	For nurse educator	For nurse administrator
• Never miss to match the patient's name and UHID on the ID band with that of medication administration record. • Always involve patient and family during medication administration. • Never prepare two patients medication together.	Train nurses on medication administration process with a stress on never taking short-cuts on medication administration protocols.	Design policy on medication administration and conduct periodic audit on the practice.

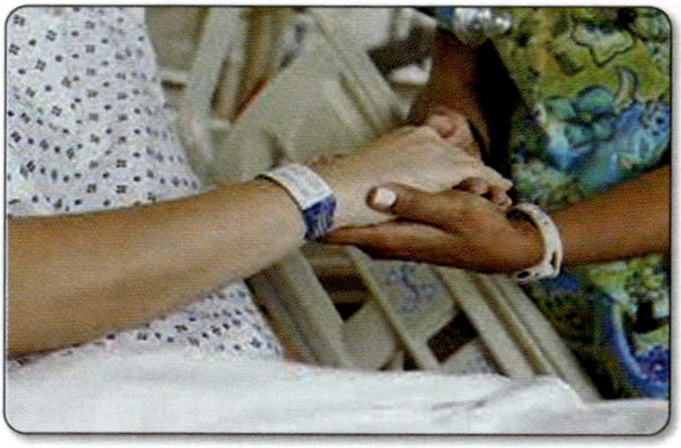

Figure 80 Confirmation of right patient by patient UHID number

Event-Based Learning Summary

This incident highlights the critical importance of patient identification in healthcare. The nurse's failure to correctly administer medications to patients with similar names emphasizes the need for strict adherence to the 'Rights of Medication Administration,' including verification of the patient's identity. All healthcare providers must ensure that they perform these checks in front of the patient, involving them in the verification process. Robust drug safety protocols that include cross-check a patient's name and unique health identifier (UHID) with the medication administration record are essential to prevent such errors. Patient identification should be assessed as a fundamental step before any procedure to enhance patient's safety. One can remember to be extra vigilant when we have similar names of patients.

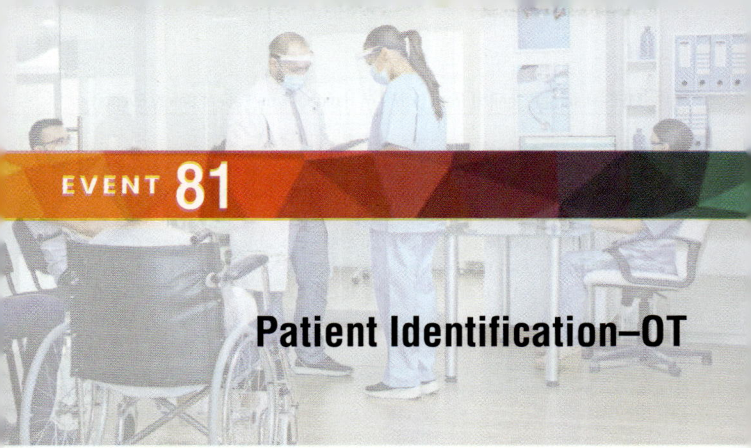

EVENT 81

Patient Identification–OT

EVENT NO.	PSE/081/092022
IPSG RELATED TO	IPSG 1 – Identify the Patient Correctly

CASE STUDY DESCRIPTION

A patient named Mr Ravi Kumar was posted for K-wiring surgery. The assigned staff nurse administered morning medication. Consents were taken and signed by the patient's relative and consultant, and the preoperative checklist was filled. The OT staff took handover from the assigned staff and the patient was mobilized to the OT preoperative area. The patient was moved to the OT after 25 minutes. During the time out, it was noted that the patient had a WRONG ID BAND. The first name was the same, but the last name/surname/ID number were different. The whole process was stopped. Mr Ravi Kumar and Mr Ravi Jain were two patients in the same unit and assigned to the same nurse, and both were posted for surgery on the same day, but the procedures were different. The patient was initially upset and furious; however, his trust was regained after an apology and explanation.

Positive Outcomes

- The time-out was carried out properly, preventing a major error.
- The hospital could regain the patient's trust.

Errors Encountered

- The process of correct patient identification had failed from the time of admission.
- Subsequently, none of the caregivers were able to notice the error indicating the fact that multiple procedures were carried out without involving the patient and verifying the information in the ID band.

Lessons Learned

For nurse	For nurse educator	For nurse administrator
• Use two identifiers to identify patients. • Involve patients in verifying their full name. • Always match patient's name and UHID number in the patient record with the information on the ID band.	• Train team on patient identification process. • Highlight the criticality of adhering to the process of patient identification through role play and scenarios. The nurses can be also warned for similar sounding and similar spelling names of patients.	• Mechanism to alert everyone when patients with similar names are admitted. • Policy can be developed to admit such patients in different rooms and assigned to different nurses.

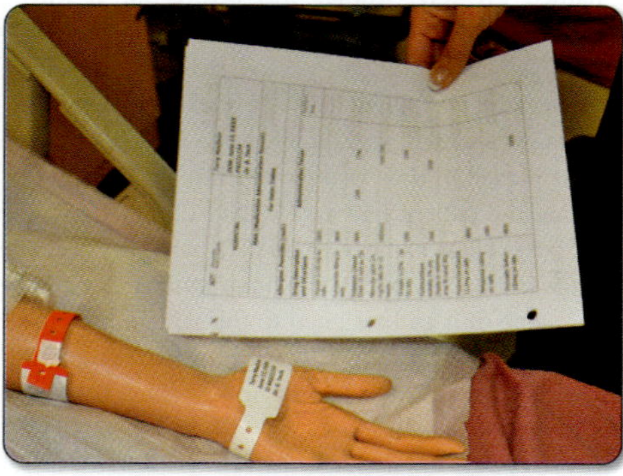

Figure 81 Patient UHID number is cross checked with file

Event-Based Learning Summary

This case underscores the critical role of patient identification from admission to the operating room. The initial error in labelling two patients with similar first names highlights the importance of robust identification protocols and compliance with safety goals. While the time-out procedure prevented a major surgical error, the incident emphasizes the need for a reliable patient identification system, from barcode generation to labelling and wristband application. Healthcare facilities should prioritize compliance with patient's safety goals and strive for continuous improvement in patient identification processes to avoid potentially dangerous consequences. Additionally, maintaining open communication with patients, offering apologies when necessary, and providing clear explanations can help rebuild patient trust after such incidents.

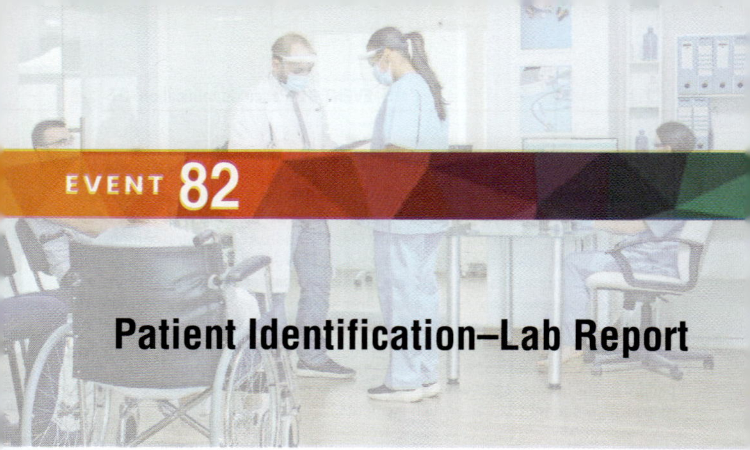

EVENT 82

Patient Identification–Lab Report

EVENT NO.	PSE/082/092022
IPSG RELATED TO	IPSG 1 – Identify the Patient Correctly

CASE STUDY DESCRIPTION

A 2-month-old preterm male baby, was admitted to the hospital on 28/6/2022 with the chief complaints of respiratory distress and reduced activity for two days. The baby was diagnosed as preterm with respiratory distress syndrome admitted to NICU-2. The baby had a history of seizure episodes managed with Syrup Levipil 12 mg.

The child developed yellow discoloration of the eyes and skin. The child seemed listless and was feeding poorly with high-pitched cries. During rounds, the consultant ordered to check the bilirubin level of child. The same investigation was asked to be done for the child in the next bed as well. The investigation result was collected through a printed copy by the shift in charge. She gave the report to one of the staff members and was told to enter it in the patient records. During rounds, the doctor asked about NICU 2 child's bilirubin report and was informed as 18 mg/dL, which was normal. But NICU in-charge was doubtful and checked the printed copy of the child's report, and it was 23 mg/dL (deciliter). Then, a neonatal specialist was called in for further treatment of the child, and the doctor asked to repeat the test for confirmation and treatment.

Positive Outcomes

- NICU in-charge was alert to check the printed copy of the child's report.
- NICU in-charge identified it at the right time, so timely treatment could be started.

Errors Encountered

- The wrong report of the child was entered in the file.
- The staff nurse failed to match name and UHID of the patient in the lab report with that of patient report.

Lessons Learned

For nurse	For nurse educator	For nurse administrator
Never fail to identify correct patient by matching the name and UHID on printed report of that patient record.	While training nurses on correct patient identification include the common identification failures by nurses.	• Periodic monitoring and review of the practice of patient identification SOPs. • Carry out random audits to check adherence to correct patient identification protocol.

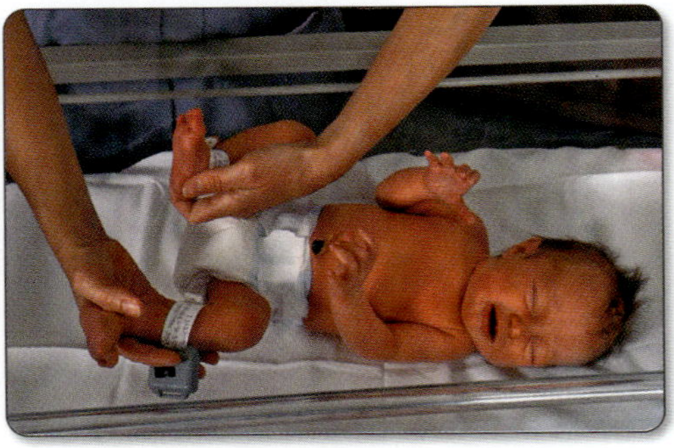

Figure 82 Using two identifiers to proceed for invasive procedure

Event-Based Learning Summary

This case underscores the critical importance of proper patient identification and documentation. The confusion and potential mismanagement of baby's condition resulted from a mix-up in patient records. The NICU in-charge's vigilance in cross-checking the printed report against her doubts prevented a medical error. It highlights the significance of a double-checking process, especially in neonatal care, where small discrepancies can have severe consequences. Healthcare providers should adhere to strict protocols for verifying and documenting patient information to prevent such incidents and ensure patient safety. Proper record-keeping, cross-verification, and diligent checks are essential components of effective neonatal care.

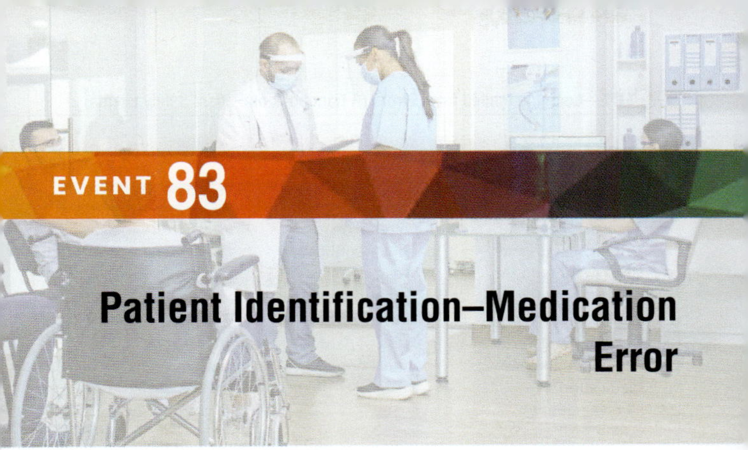

EVENT 83

Patient Identification–Medication Error

EVENT NO.	PSE/083/092022
IPSG RELATED TO	IPSG 1 – Identify the Patient Correctly

CASE STUDY DESCRIPTION

The nurse assigned in the psychiatric ward was administering routine medications using medication cards. However, the process was to counter check the doctor's order with the card. After administration of medication the nurse realized that she/he has interchanged the medications for two patients with similar names.

Positive Outcomes

- The nurse realized and admitted her mistake to the seniors.
- No adverse effect noted for the patients.

Errors Encountered

- The nurse failed to identify the correct patient by matching name and UHID in the medication card with the patients ID band.
- Two patients received wrong medications.

Lessons Learned

For nurse	For nurse educator	For nurse administrator
• Always match patient's name and UHID number in the patient record with the information on the ID band before administration of medication. • Involve patient by asking " to state your name" whenever possible.	• Train team on patient identification process. • Highlight the hidden risks of incorrect process of patient identification.	• Mechanism to alert team members on same name alerts can be developed. • "Name Alert" sticker at the door of the patients with similar names might be implemented. • Allow only privileged nurses to administer medications to patients. • Student nurses should be allowed to give medications only under strict supervision.

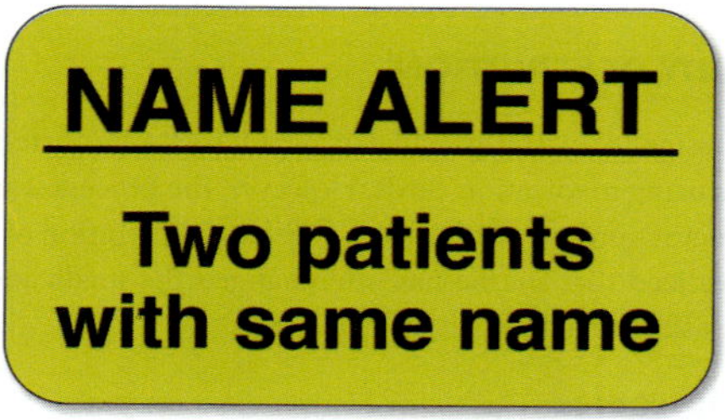

Figure 83 Signage board of name alert

Event-Based Learning Summary

This incident emphasizes the critical importance of patient identification, particularly in psychiatric wards, where medication errors can have severe consequences. The nurse's oversight in failing to double-check the patient's identity led to the administration of medication to the wrong individual. It underscores the need for strict adherence to patient identification protocols and cross-verification of medication cards, especially in settings where patients may share similar names. Healthcare providers, including trainee nurses, should be vigilant in confirming the identity of patients before administering medications to prevent errors that could jeopardize patient safety. Admitting and reporting mistakes promptly, as demonstrated by the trainee nurse, is also essential in rectifying errors and preventing adverse effects.

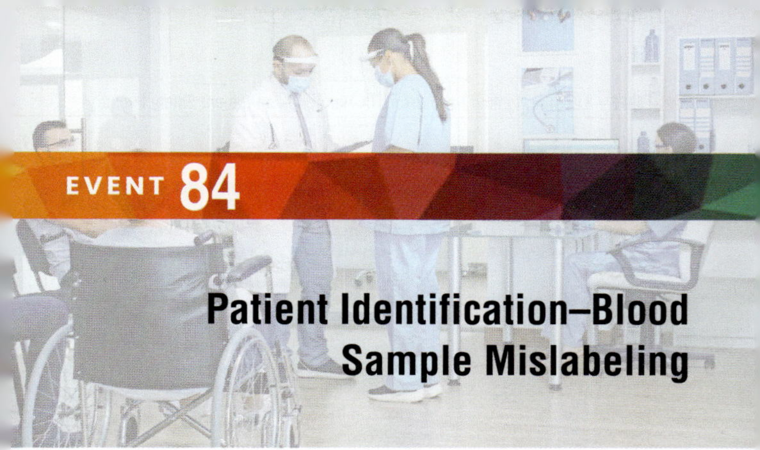

EVENT 84

Patient Identification–Blood Sample Mislabeling

EVENT NO.	PSE/084/092022
IPSG RELATED TO	IPSG 1 – Identify the Patient Correctly

CASE STUDY DESCRIPTION

A full-term mother was admitted to the hospital for safe confinement. She gave birth to a female baby through normal vaginal delivery. After delivery, there is a routine of sending cord blood samples for checking grouping and typing and the mother's blood sample for hemoglobin. The blood samples were taken and sent to the lab. But in the lab, it was found that the samples were mislabeled. The label had been interchanged between mother and baby. But before running the samples, this mistake was identified and corrected.

Positive Outcome

The mistake was identified before proceeding with the test.

Error Encountered

The labor ward nurse responsible for collecting and labeling the samples did not check properly.

Lessons Learned

For nurse	For nurse educator	For nurse administrator
• To use two patient identifiers during all the procedures. • To follow SOP on patient identification during specimen collection. • Take the sample of one patient at a time and label the container at the bedside. • Confirm the patient's name from the patient. Talk to the patient during/after the procedure taking his/her name.	• Train nurses on patient identification with reference to specimen collection. • Conduct bedside training and focus on the spot corrections. • Demonstrate proper techniques. • Use case studies and scenarios to teach.	• SOP on specimen collection to have a checkpoint on patient identification. • Conduct audits to monitor compliance. • Using technology like bar code could be useful.

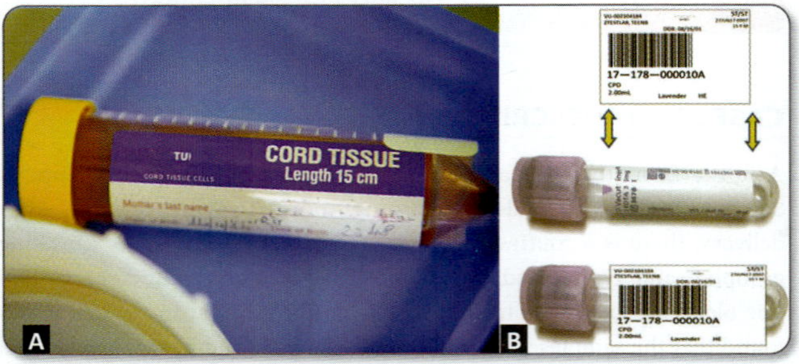

Figures 84A and B (A) Cord blood sample labeling; (B) Hemoglobin test blood sample labeling

Event-Based Learning Summary

The key takeaway from this event emphasizes the critical importance of using a multi-faceted approach to patient identification and sample labeling, even when healthcare providers are familiar with the patient. This approach should include the use of at least two identifiers, active involvement of the patient and their family, and meticulous matching of identifiers with the patient's medical record and ID band. This event serves as a reminder that human errors can occur, highlighting the need for unwavering due diligence in following established protocols consistently, each time, and every time to ensure patient safety and the accuracy of medical testing.

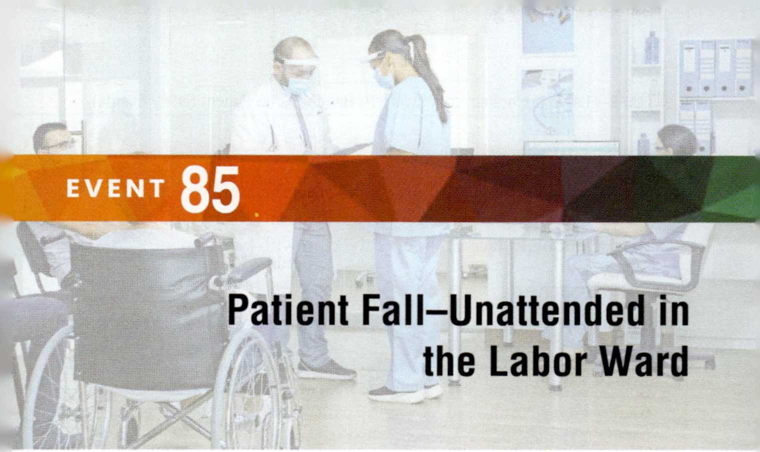

EVENT 85

Patient Fall–Unattended in the Labor Ward

EVENT NO.	PSE/085/092022
IPSG RELATED TO	IPSG 6 – Reduce the Risk of Patient Harm Resulting from Fall

CASE STUDY DESCRIPTION

26-year-old female was admitted to the labor ward after spontaneous vaginal delivery. At 8.30 am, the assigned nurse administered the routine medication to her and moved on to receive a new admission. Later, the patient went to the labor ward restroom without assistance and returned to her bed. After 10 minutes, she came to the nurses' station and asked for a sanitary napkin from the assigned nurse. While she was asking for sanitary napkins, the patient suddenly felt giddy and fell at the nurse's station. Immediately, the nurses who were nearby the nurses' station supported and assisted the patient and safely shifted the patient to her bed. After the immediate reassessment, the nurse came to know that the patient had a cut injury over the chin, with bleeding. Without delay, the staff nurses immediately informed the duty doctors and the treating team. Reassessment was done, and the treatment plan was revised. The patient's vital signs were stable.

Positive Outcome

The patient got support immediately.

Errors Encountered

- Nurses had not given postpartum fall risk education.
- The patient was not assisted to the washroom.
- The patient had a laceration over the chin with bleeding.

Lessons Learned

For nurse	For nurse educator	For nurse administrator
• Nurses must be aware of fall risk among postpartum patient regardless of the age. • The patient must be clearly explained on the risk of fall due to multiple reasons like being post general or regional anesthesia, post prolonged bed rest, post birth fatigue, blood loss, weakness and lack of sensation in lower extremities due to epidural analgesia and the side effects of medications received. • Educate family members to be with the patient while ambulating. • Nurses must do a thorough fall risk assessment before allowing the patient to ambulate.	• To train nurses on patient fall assessment and prevention, especially in pregnant and postpartum mothers. • Train nurses on fall risk assessment and precaution in special category. • Review incidents and share them with the staff along with the root cause and the corrective-preventive actions taken.	• To devise interventions depending on the risk level of the patient. • Conduct safety rounds. • Ensure a safe environment.

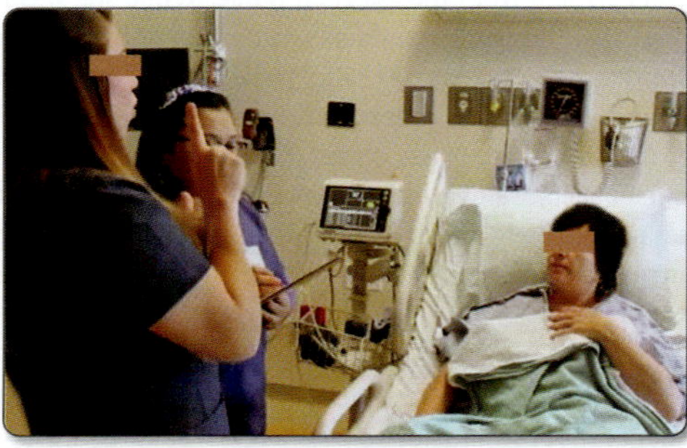

Figure 85 Nurse along with interpreter performing periodic fall assessment

Event-Based Learning Summary

This event underscores the significance of personalized patient care, especially for young patients who may be prone to falls due to their unique medical conditions and physiological changes. Nurses must comprehensively understand each patient's individual needs and provide tailored instructions. In the case of pregnant and postpartum patients, the hemodynamic changes they experience emphasize the necessity of clear communication with patients about why precautions are essential during their movements. The key takeaway from this incident is that patient safety can be greatly enhanced through customized care and effective communication to prevent falls and ensure the well-being of all patients, regardless of age.

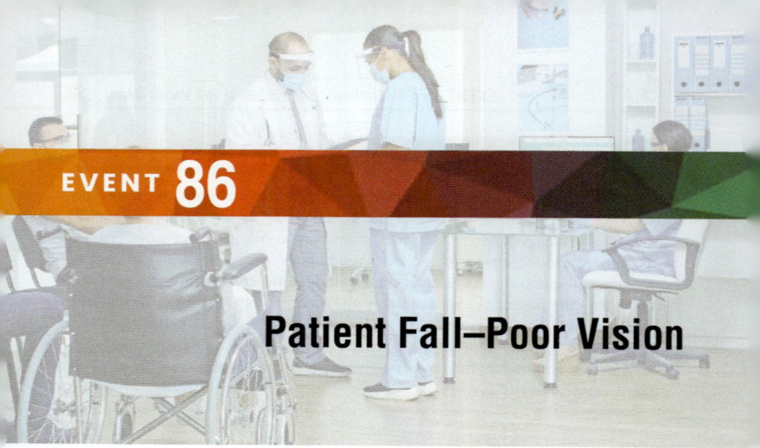

EVENT 86

Patient Fall–Poor Vision

EVENT NO.	PSE/086/092022
IPSG RELATED TO	IPSG 6 – Reduce the Risk of Patient Harm Resulting from Fall

CASE STUDY DESCRIPTION

Mr Farhad, a 70-year-old patient from another country, was admitted for chronic liver disease. He had a guardian from India and no relatives who accompanied him. The relatives were going to come later. The patient couldn't speak or understand English. In his initial assessment, the nurse had missed understanding that the patient had difficulty with his vision and used the stick for ambulation. The nurse explained that they needed to call for assistance, using the call bell, and not to walk without help. On the third day, at noon, the patient went to the washroom without assistance, and sustained a fall at the washroom entrance. The patient was attended to immediately, lifted, and taken to the bed, monitored vital signs, and a physical examination was performed. It was challenging to get all the patient's subjective complaints and how exactly the fall happened because of the language barrier. The duty doctor and registrar examined the patient, and no external injuries were found. The nurse noted that the patient was drowsy the next day and did not respond well to her questions. This was escalated to the consultant, a neuro opinion was obtained, and CT revealed an internal brain hemorrhage due to the head injury during the fall. The patient had to be admitted to neuro-ICU and taken for surgery after the relatives had come over.

Positive Outcome

The neurological deterioration in the patient after the fall was identified by the assigned nurse promptly.

Errors Encountered

- During the initial assessment critical assessment questions were missed (vision, hearing, stick for walking).
- The preventive measures were not explained in an understandable language to the patient.
- The sequence of the fall and the injuries were not ascertained due to the language barrier.
- Failure to identify the head injury during first physical examination after the fall.

Lessons Learned

For nurse	For nurse educator	For nurse administrator
• Periodic fall assessment and education to the patient and family. • Nurses must request for translator when they identify language barrier. • Nurses must take cue from aids the patient may bring along (walking stick, hearing aids, glasses, etc.) and ask relevant questions to plan appropriate nursing care.	• Train nurses on patient fall assessment and prevention. • Emphasize on different category of patients who are at risk for fall and the critical role of patient understanding their role in preventing falls. • Educate nurses to ask for translators whenever there is a language barrier.	• Device intervention and support to personalize fall risk assessment and interventions. • Recommend to have translators whenever they have language barrier to have right things communicated to the patients.

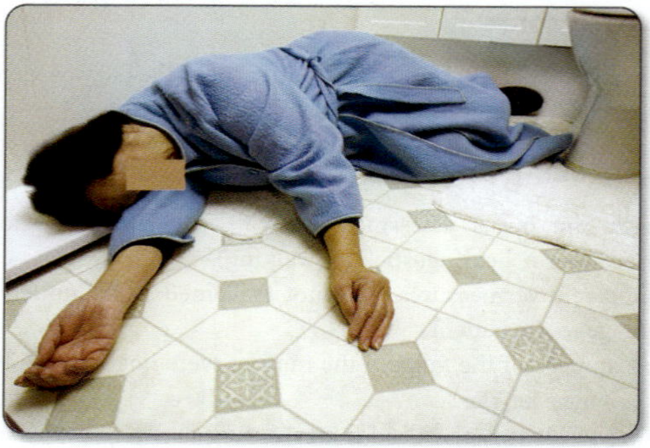

Figure 86 Patient falling in bathroom

Event-Based Learning Summary

This incident highlights the importance of comprehensive initial assessments, particularly for vulnerable patients over the age of 65. It is crucial to inquire about various factors, including vision, hearing, mobility with aids, and other potential fall risk indicators. When language barriers exist, healthcare providers should proactively use translation services or employ culturally sensitive communication strategies to ensure patients and their guardians fully understand preventive measures. Furthermore, clear and understandable explanations about the importance of using call bells and seeking assistance must be provided.

Effective interdisciplinary collaboration, involving nurses and clinicians, is essential in promptly identifying and addressing fall-related incidents. Continuous monitoring and examination for external injuries are essential in such cases. The case emphasizes that even minor falls should not be underestimated, as comprehensive assessment and communication are critical in ensuring patient safety and timely interventions.

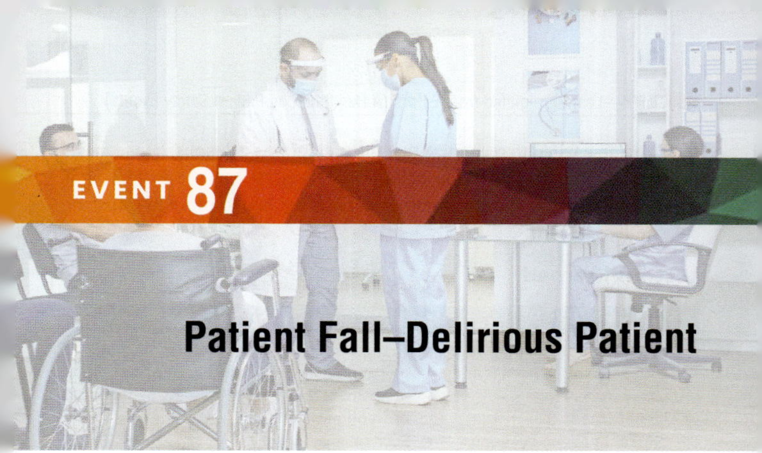

EVENT 87

Patient Fall–Delirious Patient

EVENT NO.	PSE/087/092022
IPSG RELATED TO	IPSG 6 – Reduce the Risk of Patient Harm Resulting from Fall

CASE STUDY DESCRIPTION

At 12:30 am, Mr Vishal was transferred from neuro high dependency unit (HDU). He was conscious but had delirium. His daughter and the HDU staff nurse accompanied him to the private ward. The ward staff gave room orientation, use of call bell, side rails, etc. Around 4 am, there was a call bell from this patient's room. The nurse immediately attended to it; the patient wanted to go to the washroom to pass the motion. The nurse insisted that he was wearing diapers and could pass the motion in the diaper and explained that he is restricted in moving out of the bed. At the same time, the nurse was required to shift another patient to dialysis. And she moved out. After a few minutes, there was a loud noise, and that patient's relative started calling. The patient jumped out of bed and experienced a fall. He was immediately seen by doctor, underwent some investigations, and was shifted to neuro ICU again.

Positive Outcome

None.

Errors Encountered

- The timing of the transfer was inappropriate.
- The nurse failed to offer a bedpan instead of insisting on using a diaper.

- The nurse failed to recognize that the patient was delirious, hence may not comprehend and follow her advice.
- The nurse failed to call in another nurse if she had to move to transfer another patient.

Lessons Learned

For nurse	For nurse educator	For nurse administrator
• Periodic fall assessment and education to the patient and family. • Identify the specific risk in different patient. (Delirious patient) • Inform doctor for appropriate intervention for a delirious patient and never leave such patient specially when they ask to go to the washroom. • Take time to communicate with patients and relatives and have another nurse be available if the nurse need to move out.	• To train nurses on patient fall assessment and prevention. • Such case studies must be discussed during training so that nurses understand the different reasons in the different categories of patient resulting in fall.	Device intervention and support to personalize fall risk assessment and interventions.

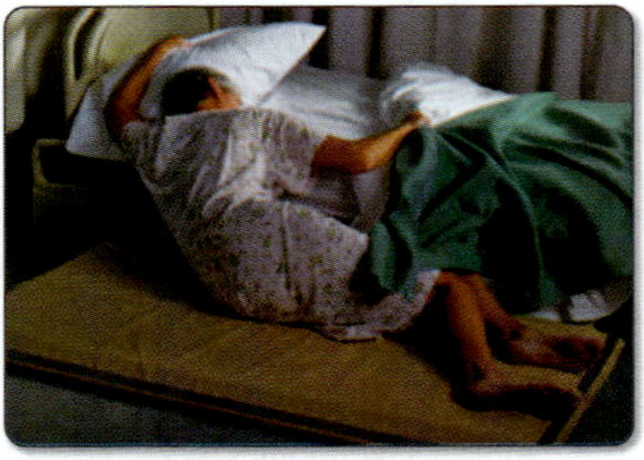

Figure 87 Patient fall

Event-Based Learning Summary

The incident highlights the importance of patient transfers, especially for those with cognitive impairments like delirium. Timing is crucial, and nurses must assess each patient's unique needs, offering suitable solutions, and closely supervising to prevent falls. Educating both patients and their families on fall prevention is paramount. Adequate staffing and delegation ensure that patient care remains a top priority, and seeking assistance from colleagues when needed is a crucial safety measure.

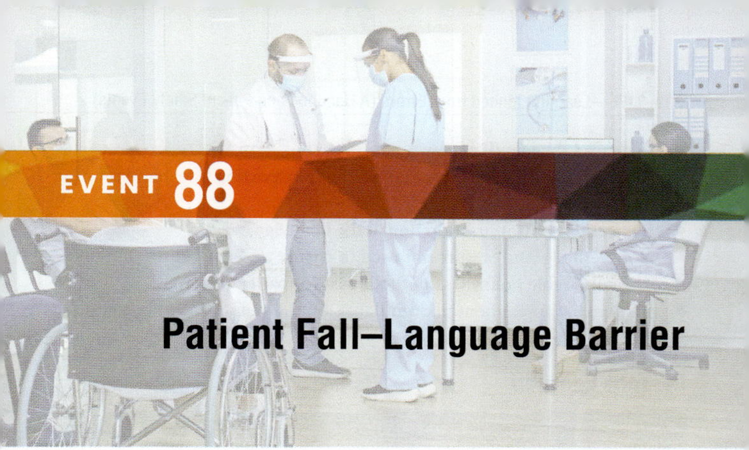

EVENT 88

Patient Fall–Language Barrier

EVENT NO.	PSE/088/092022
IPSG RELATED TO	IPSG 6 – Reduce the Risk of Patient Harm Resulting from Fall

CASE STUDY DESCRIPTION

Mr Srinivas Raghavan, a 91-year-old male patient, was admitted to the surgical ward with pain in the abdomen. Abdomen sonography revealed right side inguinal hernia with long segment inflammatory bowel wall thickening. Since there were lot of air shadows, CT scan was recommended to rule out bowel perforation. The housekeeping attendant took the patient to the CT scan room. He parked the wheelchair beside the CT scan table and told the patient not to get up. He told the patient that he would help the patient to the table. But the patient had a language issue, so he got up from the wheelchair and, due to imbalance, fell down. The patient had a minor laceration on the left elbow. Later on, it was found that the patient had sustained a fracture.

Positive Outcome

None.

Errors Encountered

- The patient had a minor laceration on the left elbow.
- The patient got a left intertrochanteric (IT) fracture.

- Increased the length of stay.
- A safety belt was not applied while transporting the patient in a wheelchair.
- Ineffective communication due to the language barrier.
- Non-verbal gestures were not used to ensure understanding.
- The vulnerable policy was not followed for patient safety.
- Incomplete assessment and guidance by the nurse while shifting the patient.

Lessons Learned

For nurse	For nurse educator	For nurse administrator
• Periodic fall assessment and education to the patient and family. • Nurses should ask for translators. • Nurses must assess the patient for fall risk keeping in mind all aspects of individual patients. (91-year old possibly with an acute abdomen must have been shifted on a stretcher with a nurse).	• Train nurses on fall risk assessment and precaution in special category. • Such case studies must be discussed during training so that nurses understand the different reasons in the different categories of patient resulting in fall.	• To devise interventions depending on the risk level of the patient. • Devise intervention and support to personalize fall risk assessment and interventions. • Facilitate having appropriate translators to respond to calls from nurses when they identify language barrier.

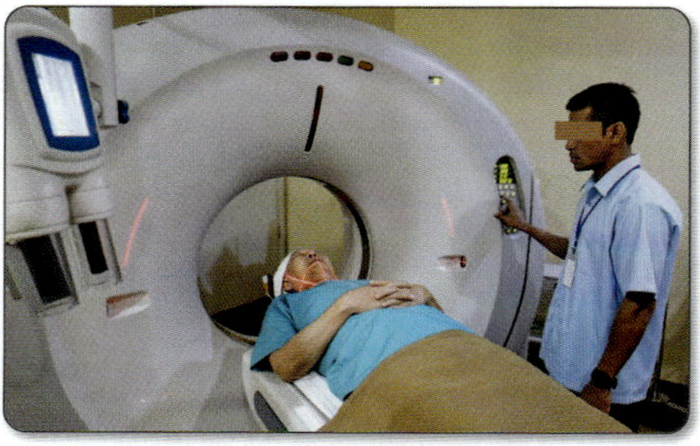

Figure 88 Patient for CT scan

Event-Based Learning Summary

This incident emphasizes the critical importance of effective communication and understanding when caring for patients, particularly in cases involving language barriers. Nonverbal communication, like gestures and clear instructions, is essential to ensure patient safety. Furthermore, nurses must make diligent efforts to find an interpreter when necessary, recognizing that a 91-year-old patient is at a higher risk for accidents and misunderstandings. Adhering to protocols, such as using safety belts during patient transport, is crucial to prevent incidents. This event also highlights the need for proper training and protocols for attendants to ensure patient safety during transfers.

This incident also emphasizes the critical need for nurses to assess individual patients for fall risk during transfers and delegate only if the safety is ensured.

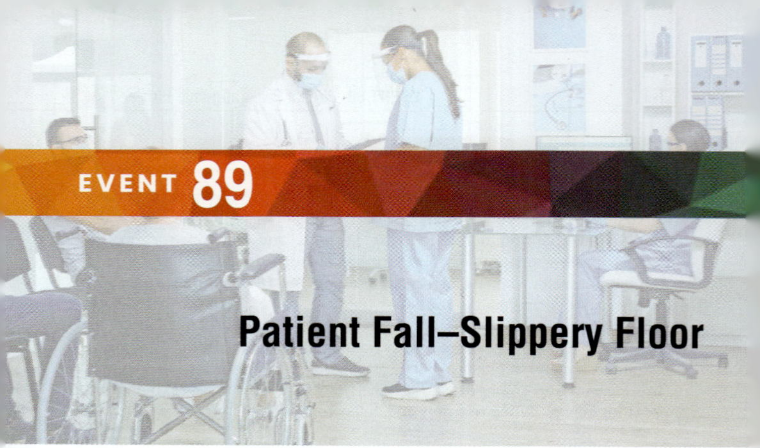

EVENT 89

Patient Fall–Slippery Floor

EVENT NO.	PSE/089/092022
IPSG RELATED TO	IPSG 6 – Reduce the Risk of Patient Harm Resulting from Fall

CASE STUDY DESCRIPTION

Mr Saurabh, a 68-year-old gentleman, got admitted to the Gastro ward with the diagnosis of chronic peptic ulcer. The patient had history of hearing loss. The assigned nurse did not identify this sensory impairment in the initial patient assessment. The patient went to the washroom in the night without attendant and fell down on the floor where water was spilled. He slipped and fell down, and could not stand; he had severe pain in the left hip region. The patient was attended to immediately, lifted, and taken to bed. The duty doctor examined the patient, and an urgent X-ray was taken; which revealed a fracture on the neck of the femur. He was transferred to the Ortho department and planned for surgery.

Positive Outcome

None.

Errors Encountered

- Inaccurate and incomplete initial assessment.
- Inadequate supervision by the senior staff.
- Due to hearing impairment, all education/explanation might not have been understood by the patient.

- The patient's attendant was not briefed on the fall risk and what safety measures needed to be observed.

Lessons Learned

For nurse	For nurse educator	For nurse administrator
• Periodic fall assessment and education to the patient and family. • Never miss to assess for any sensory impairment during initial assessment. • After educating patient and attendant about the fall risk and prevention strategies, never miss to use teach-back technique to ensure understanding.	• Train nurses on patient fall assessment and prevention. • Discuss such scenarios during training to emphasize the importance of complete and accurate initial assessment, to individualize patient education on fall prevention.	• To devise interventions depending on the risk level of the patient. • Safety measures when in the toilet (putting the lights on, checking if the floor is wet, if wet, asking for cleaning) should have been emphasized. • Involve front-line nurses in root cause analysis of adverse events and initiate learning sessions based on such events.

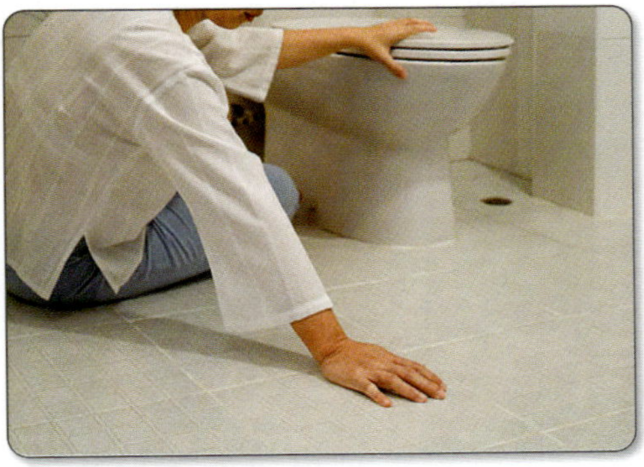

Figure 89 Patient falling in bathroom

Event-Based Learning Summary

This incident emphasizes that accidents can occur due to unfamiliarity with hospital settings, even among patients who may not be considered vulnerable. Patients must be made aware of the potential risks within the hospital environment to ensure their safety. Additionally, it highlights the critical role of thorough and competent patient assessments, particularly when dealing with new or inexperienced staff members. Inadequate assessment, lack of supervision, and the absence of clear communication can lead to critical incidents like patient falls. Healthcare professionals must consider a patient's specific needs and conditions, such as hearing impairment, to ensure proper education and safety measures. It also underscores the importance of briefing attendants on fall risks and preventive measures, especially when patients are at risk due to medical conditions.

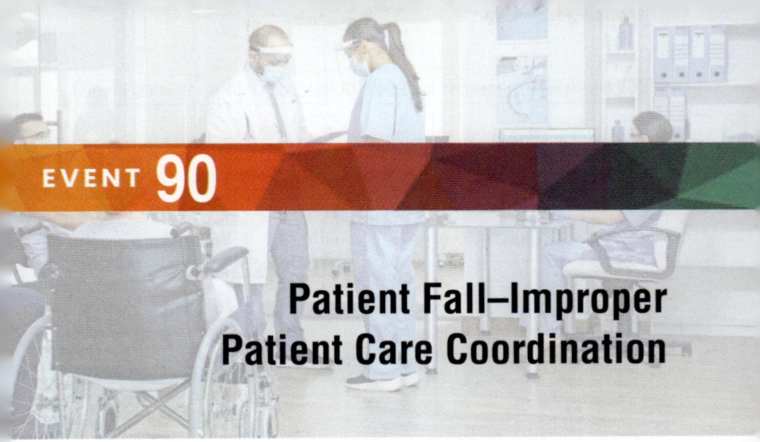

EVENT 90

Patient Fall–Improper Patient Care Coordination

EVENT NO.	PSE/090/092022
IPSG RELATED TO	IPSG 6 – Reduce the Risk of Patient Harm Resulting from Fall

CASE STUDY DESCRIPTION

The doctor received a call from the nursing supervisor that one of the patients had sustained a fall and got a cut wound on his forehead. When doctor asked for the reason for the fall it was informed that during sponge bath patient sustained a fall when he was turned to the side. Further inquiry revealed that the patient was on an air mattress, the height of which was same as the side rails. So when the patient was turned the housekeeping staff could not balance the patient weight leading to the fall of the patient. He hit his head on the locker kept at the side and sustained an injury.

Positive Outcome

Fortunately, the patient did not have any major injury.

Errors Encountered

- The nurse had not deflated the air mattress placed on the patient's bed.
- The nurse had not warned the housekeeping staff on the risk and the safety precautions.

Lessons Learned

For nurse	For nurse educator	For nurse administrator
• Always do patient safety assessment before starting any procedure. • Ask for adequate help before starting any procedure. • Take help from companions. • Deflate the air mattress before rolling the patient over for procedures.	Train nurses on fall prevention when turning and mobilizing patients including checking all the equipment and devices attached.	• To devise interventions depending on the risk level of the patient. • Involve front-line nurses in root cause analysis of adverse events and initiate learning sessions based on such events.

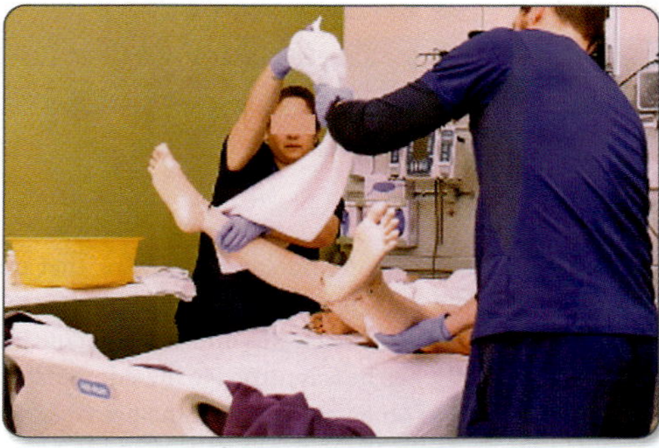

Figure 90 Nurse turning the patient for back care with housekeeping staff

Event-Based Learning Summary

This incident highlights the significance of proper patient care coordination to prevent falls and injuries in healthcare settings. Inadequate communication and teamwork among healthcare staff can lead to unfortunate incidents like patient falls. In this case, the failure to coordinate between the nurse and the housekeeping person, who was assisting with patient care, resulted in the patient falling and sustaining an injury. It is crucial for healthcare professionals to work together efficiently and communicate effectively to ensure patient safety. In addition, ensuring that medical equipment, like air mattress, is properly managed and used can prevent accidents and potential injuries to patients. Proper patient care coordination can help avoid such incidents and promote a safe healthcare environment.

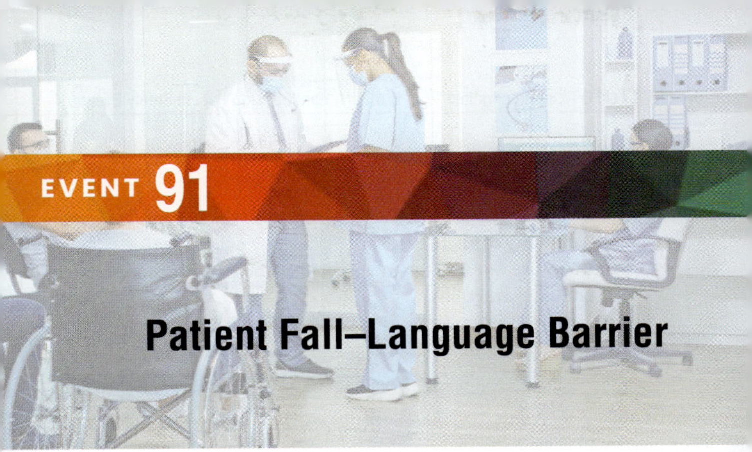

EVENT 91

Patient Fall–Language Barrier

EVENT NO.	PSE/091/092022
IPSG RELATED TO	IPSG 6 – Reduce the Risk of Patient Harm Resulting from Fall

CASE STUDY DESCRIPTION

Mr Ganesh Sridhar, a 66-year-old male patient, was hospitalized for cataract surgery. The patient could not speak and understand Tamil and his mother tongue was Telugu. In addition, the patient had difficulty seeing through the right eye due to surgery. The nurse gave all instructions to the available attendant. On the second day patient went to washroom without any assistance and sustained the fall in the washroom. As the nurse was available at the room for medication administration, immediate help was provided. On examination, there was no external injuries. Because of the language barrier it could not be ascertained how he fell in the washroom.

Positive Outcomes

None.

Errors Encountered

- Incomplete assessment and patient education.
- Failure to identify the increased risk of fall in the patient due to poor understanding of instructions.
- Failure to use a translator to ensure that the patient understand fall prevention instructions.

Lessons Learned

For nurse	For nurse educator	For nurse administrator
• Nurses must do a complete fall prevention assessment and individualize the prevention strategies. • Whenever there is language barrier ask for translator to ensure full understanding of the fall prevention instructions.	Train nurses on patient fall-risk assessment and prevention.	• To devise interventions depending on the risk level of the patient. • It is recommended to have appropriate translators to respond to calls from nurses when they identify language barrier.

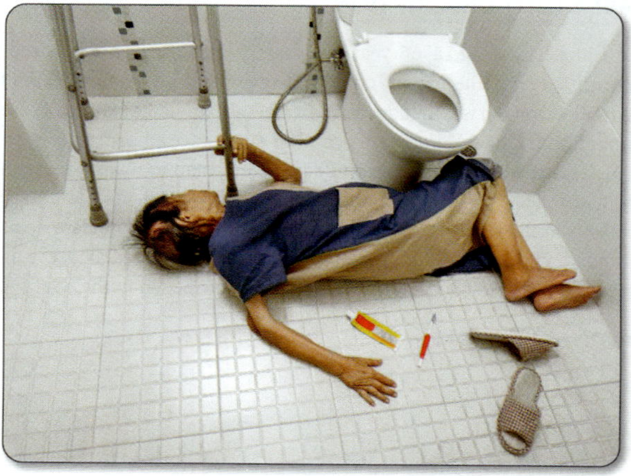

Figure 91 Patient falling and getting injured in bathroom

Event-Based Learning Summary

This incident underscores the critical role of effective communication and patient education, especially when language barriers are present. In cases like Mr. Ganesh Sridhar's, who could not communicate in the local language and had impaired vision due to eye surgery, it is vital to ensure that patients understand how to seek assistance and use call bells for help, particularly during activities like ambulation. Proper patient education can prevent accidents and falls. In this case, the failure to address the language barrier and provide clear instructions led to the patient attempting to use the washroom without assistance, resulting in a fall.

Healthcare providers need to identify and address language barriers promptly. Employ interpreters or alternative communication methods to ensure that patients comprehend critical instructions. Patient safety is enhanced when patients understand how to seek help and when healthcare providers prioritize clear communication in diverse linguistic and cultural settings.

This incident serves as a reminder that healthcare professionals should adapt their care and communication to each patient's unique needs, particularly when language barriers and impairments are factors.

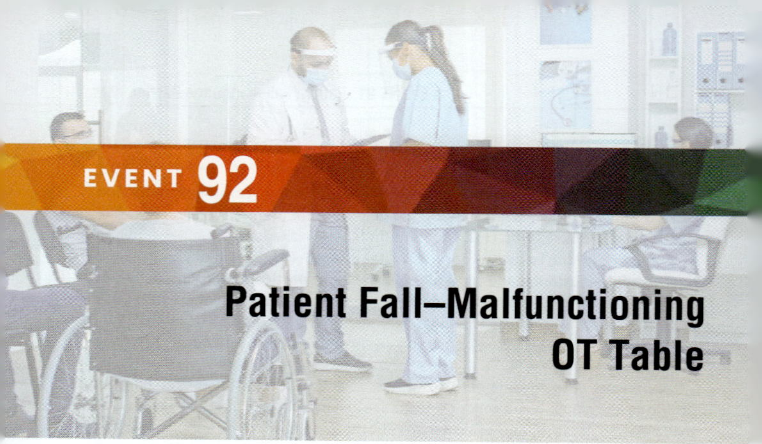

EVENT 92

Patient Fall–Malfunctioning OT Table

EVENT NO.	PSE/092/092022
IPSG RELATED TO	IPSG 6 – Reduce the Risk of Patient Harm Resulting from Fall

CASE STUDY DESCRIPTION

Mr Abhishek Kumar was in the OT for surgery. After giving spinal anesthesia while positioning the patient, the OT table got tilted toward the leg end, and the patient slipped in that direction. But fortunately, OT staff was alert and prevented the patient from falling, although the patient's foot touched the floor. Since the patient was conscious, counseling was done, he was shifted to another table, and surgery was conducted. It was found that four nut bolts of the OT table had come out, resulting in this incident.

Positive Outcome

The staff was vigilant toward the patient and prevented the fall from the OT table.

Errors Encountered

The defect of the OT Table was not detected indicating failure to check the safe functioning of OT table. This also indicates failure of periodic preventive maintenance.

Lessons Learned

For nurse	For nurse educator	For nurse administrator
• Daily checking of critical equipment. • Ensure procedure readiness. • Verify regular preventive maintenance of all OT equipment.	• Train all OT nurses on safe practices in the OT as all the patient's are vulnerable to fall from a narrow OT table. • Discuss the criticality of all OT equipment before shifting the patient to OT table.	• Ensure OT nurses and other OT staff receive training on safe practices to prevent patient fall in OT. • Safety checklist can be used to ensure compliance to do the safe practices.

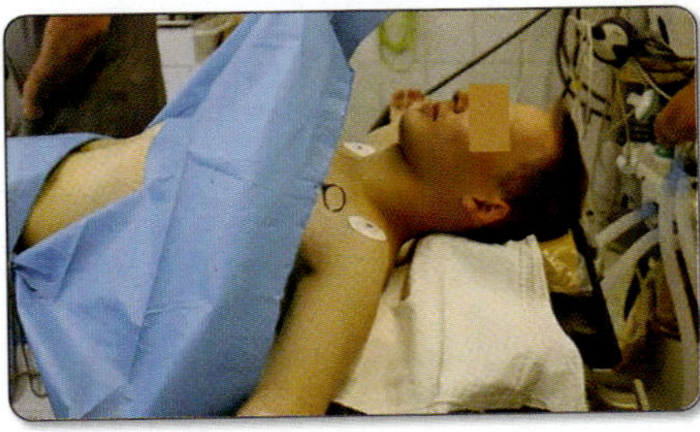

Figure 92 Patient is on OT table

Event-Based Learning Summary

This incident highlights the critical importance of maintaining and regularly inspecting medical equipment for patient safety. In Mr Abhishek Kumar's case, the OT table malfunctioned during surgery, causing the patient to slip. Fortunately, the operating room staff reacted quickly to prevent the fall and ensured the patient's well-being.

To enhance patient safety, healthcare facilities should implement robust equipment maintenance and inspection protocols. Routine checks can help identify and address equipment issues before they lead to patient harm. In this case, the failure to identify the OT table's defect prior to the procedure underscored the need for rigorous equipment maintenance and safety checks to prevent adverse events.

Healthcare providers must prioritize the safety of patients by ensuring that all medical equipment are in proper working condition. Addressing equipment malfunctions promptly and implementing preventive measures are essential to maintain the trust and safety of patients in healthcare settings.

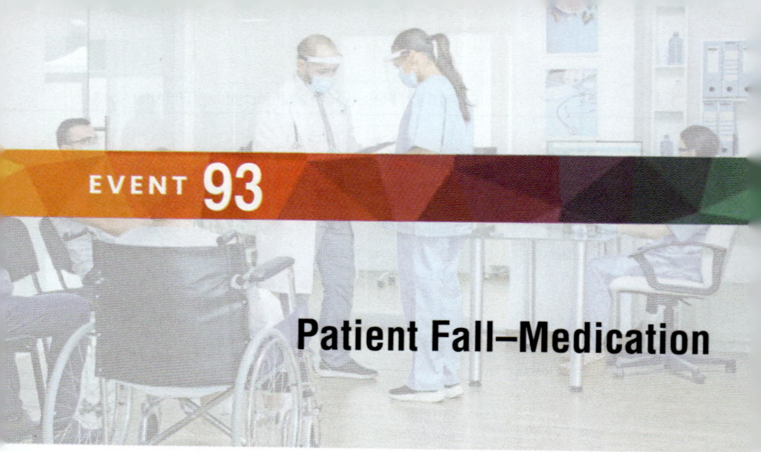

EVENT 93

Patient Fall–Medication

EVENT NO.	PSE/093/092022
IPSG RELATED TO	IPSG 6 – Reduce the Risk of Patient Harm Resulting from Fall

CASE STUDY DESCRIPTION

Mr Bheem Singh was admitted to the medical ward with the complaints of uncontrolled hypertension. The patient was newly-started with Tab. Labetalol, which the assigned nurse administered. After 2 hours, suddenly the patient fell down while going to the bathroom. He was conscious. Immediately the patient got back to bed. A physical examination revealed no external injuries. Patient verbalized, he felt giddiness and light-headedness and fell down. Vital parameters were normal and CT brain was taken to rule out internal hemorrhages, CT brain showed no abnormal findings.

Positive Outcome

None.

Errors Encountered

- Failure to anticipate the potential for Orthostatic Hypotension after the first dose of Tab Labetalol, a potent high alert anti-hypertensive drug.
- Failure to educate the patient how to prevent orthostatic hypotension.

Lessons Learned

For nurse	For nurse educator	For nurse administrator
• Learn about the drugs and their side effects before administering medications. • If a nurse is new to a drug, ensure that you learn the action and side effects from doctor/seniors. • Drug reference book or online resources can also be referred. Labetalol being a high risk medicine must be supervised by another nurse. • Teaching patient on side effect and the steps to prevent orthostatic hypotension is critical in cardiovascular drugs.	Educate nurses on drugs that can increase the risk of fall in patients.	Ensure that the fall risk assessment tool being used in the hospital must have the evidence -based list of medications that increase the risk of patient fall.

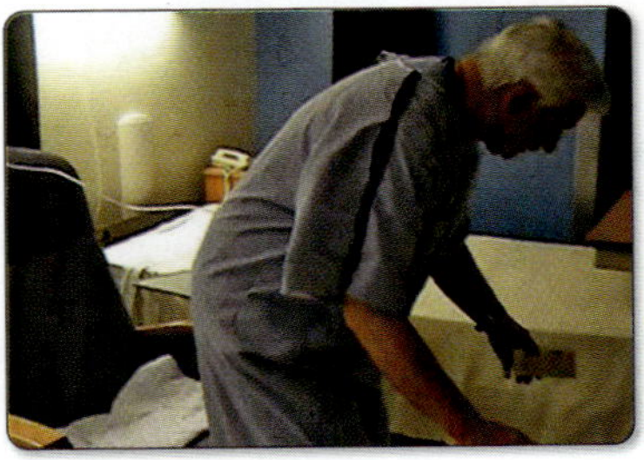

Figure 93 Patient fall

Event-Based Learning Summary

This incident emphasizes the importance of medication education and fall risk assessment in patient safety. A patient, newly prescribed Tab. Labetalol for hypertension, experienced a fall shortly after taking the medication. While immediate post-fall care was provided, and the patient had no external injuries, there was a significant lapse in medication safety, as patient education regarding potential side effects was missing. Anticipating and addressing fall risk factors and conducting ongoing risk assessments were also overlooked.

To enhance patient safety, healthcare providers must prioritize thorough patient education about medication side effects and fall risk factors. Regular fall risk assessments, particularly when patients start new medications or experience changes in their conditions, are essential. Implementing preventive measures and safety protocols can play a critical role in reducing fall-related incidents.

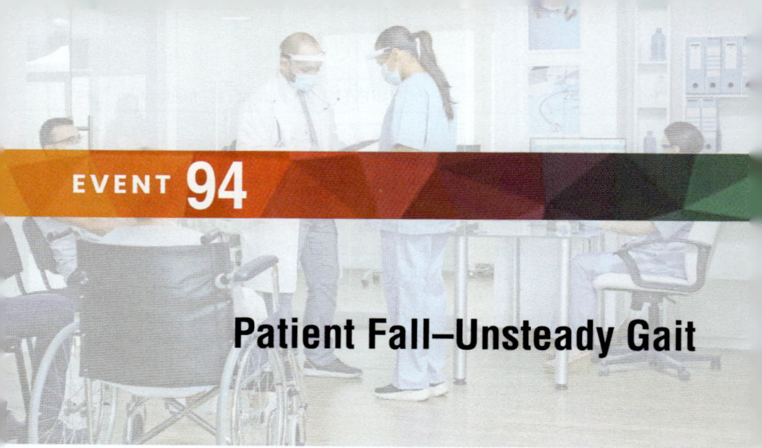

EVENT 94

Patient Fall–Unsteady Gait

EVENT NO.	PSE/094/092022
IPSG RELATED TO	IPSG 6 – Reduce the Risk of Patient Harm Resulting from Fall

CASE STUDY DESCRIPTION

A 40-year-old patient was admitted with end-stage liver cirrhosis. Though on palliative care, he was alert, oriented, and conscious. The patient was on fall precaution due to his unsteady gait. The patient pressed the call bell during the night and requested a urinal. The urinal was provided, and the patient asked the nurse to continue with her work and that he would call her once he voided. The nurse moved to the other patient. Within a few minutes, there was a loud noise. When the nurse reached the patient side, he was on the floor. The incident report was made, and the protocol was followed.

Positive Outcome

On post-fall assessment, the patient did not have any injury.

Error Encountered

Failure to anticipate that the patient with unsteady gait must not be left alone standing for voiding.

Lessons Learned

For nurse	For nurse educator	For nurse administrator
• Individualize fall prevention strategies for patients based on their diagnosis, fall risk assessment and medication. • Do not leave patients alone standing when they have history of unsteady gait. • Even if the patient asks the nurse to come back later, the nurse must be able to educate the patient about the need for having someone to support while standing up to pass urine.	• Train nurses on fall risk assessment and prevention. • Discuss such cases with the nurses to know that even younger patients be at risk of fall.	• Ensure periodic audits on fall risk assessment done by nurses. • Plan to discuss the audit results and facilitate learning from such events.

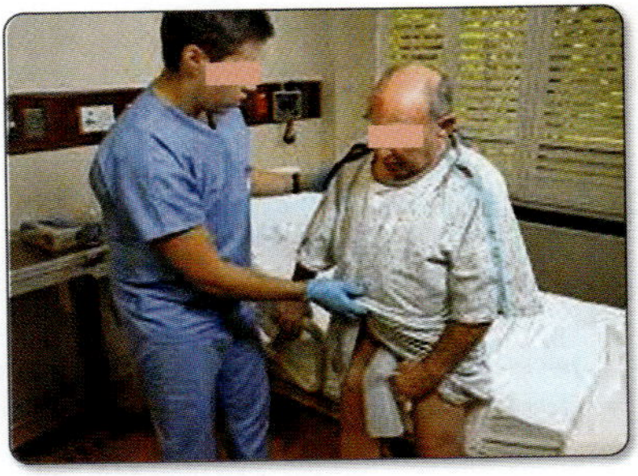

Figure 94 Assisting male patient in voiding urine

Event-Based Learning Summary

Knowing patients well is paramount for nurses, and it extends beyond just medical data. It involves understanding their preferences and needs. In the case of a 40-year-old gentleman admitted with end-stage liver cirrhosis, he was on fall precautions due to an unsteady gait. When he requested a urinal, the nurse provided it but failed to ask if he was comfortable using it in bed. The incident report showed that the patient had fallen. This incident emphasizes that even when patients are on fall precautions and side rails are in place, it does not guarantee their safety. Effective communication at every step is essential. Nurses should remind patients that they are there to help, inquire about their preferences, and ensure that all safety measures are tailored to the individual, thus preventing such incidents.

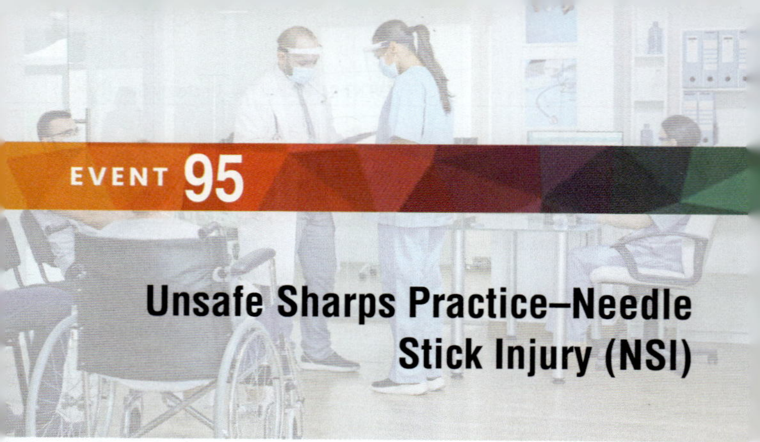

EVENT 95

Unsafe Sharps Practice–Needle Stick Injury (NSI)

EVENT NO.	PSE/095/092022
IPSG RELATED TO	None

CASE STUDY DESCRIPTION

Ms Sophia, a staff nurse working in general ward B, had six patients assigned. She was called by one patient who complained of pain at the IV site, and she assessed that there was a need for reinserting another cannula. She prepared the tray and performed the procedure, and after completion of the procedure, she handed over her procedure tray with the needle, gloves, gauze, paper, etc., to the GDA for disposal. The GDA, while segregating the waste, sustained a needle stick injury.

Positive Outcome

None.

Error Encountered

The GDA sustained a needle stick injury.

Lessons Learned

For nurse	For nurse educator	For nurse administrator
• To segregate and discard the waste at the source of generation. • Not to transfer sharps. • Carry a small Puncture Proof Container in IV cannulation tray and discard the needle in the PPC directly. • Use safety devices. • Use proper techniques. • Wear protective equipment. • Attend trainings. • Report incidents.	• Educate nurses on NSI prevention. • Teach nurses the proper work practices that help prevent needlestick injuries, such as safe handling of sharps, no recapping of needles, and avoiding disassembling sharps. • Emphasize not to delegate segregation of sharps waste to another personnel.	• Portable sharps containers can be made available for performing bedside procedures, where needles/sharps can be discarded at the source. • Implement sharp safety protocols. • Ensure regular safety trainings are conducted. • Monitor compliance by conducting audits.

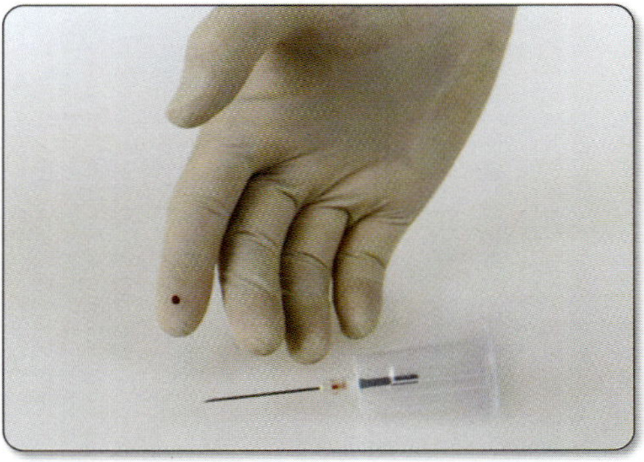

Figure 95 Needle stick injury from IV cannula needle

Event-Based Learning Summary

This incident emphasizes the fundamental principle of biomedical waste disposal, which emphasizes that waste generators should be responsible for segregating and disposing of waste at the source. In this case, the involvement of the General Duty Assistant (GDA) in disposing of sharps waste was inappropriate, as they do not generate sharps waste themselves. It is important to note that despite well-known procedures and guidelines, some nurses may engage in risky behaviors that put others at risk of acquiring diseases from bloodborne pathogens. A professional nurse should prioritize the safety of both themselves and their coworkers by strictly adhering to safe disposal practices.

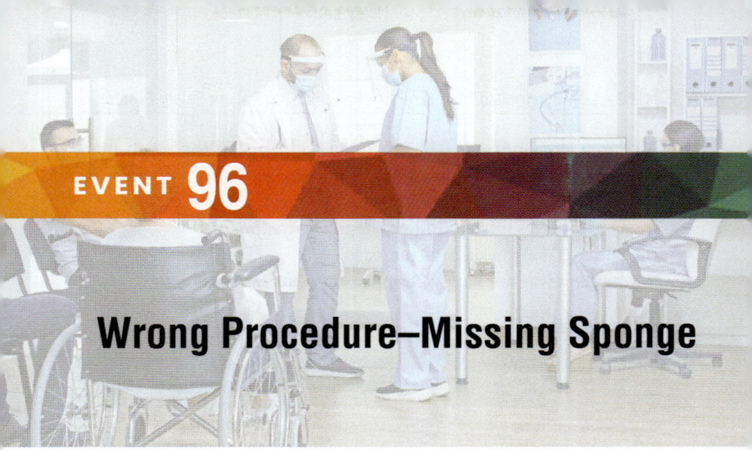

EVENT 96

Wrong Procedure–Missing Sponge

EVENT NO.	PSE/096/092022
IPSG RELATED TO	IPSG 4 – Ensure Correct Site, Correct Procedure, Correct Patient Surgery

CASE STUDY DESCRIPTION

In the operation theater during surgery scrub nurse was relieved for meal break and the relieving scrub nurse did not take over the counts as she felt that she was relieving for 30 minutes only. By the time the closure was initiated, the first scrub nurse was still not back from the meal break. During the wound closure, the circulating nurse found that one X-ray detectable sponge was missing. A search was done in the patient's wound, in the dustbins of that OT, but it was not found. An X-ray of the patient's abdomen was taken on the table, but no sponge was found in the scan. Later the surgeon concluded the surgery, and the wound was closed.

Positive Outcomes

- The missing count was informed to the surgeon.
- The on-table X-ray was taken.

Errors Encountered

- The sponge count at every stage of transition was missing.
- The scrub nurse handing over and taking over missed the seriousness of counting the sponge during the change in scrub nurses.

- The circulatory nurse was not firm enough to stop the scrub nurse when the handover was not done.
- The patient was unnecessarily exposed to X-ray.
- The OT time was wasted finding the missing sponge.
- The patient's anesthesia time increased.
- The surgeon was not happy despite a very successful surgery.

Lessons Learned

For nurse	For nurse educator	For nurse administrator
• The counts must be taken before the skin closure and also when there is a change in the scrub nurse. • Diligent adherence to the surgical safety checklist. • Use effective communication skills with assertiveness to point out errors.	• Train nurses on surgical safety checklist with emphasis on counts verification. • Provide an overview of the counting process. • Demonstrate the process. • Provide hands-on training. • Train by means of role-play enacting various situations that can occur. • Provide training on critical safety aspects.	• Conduct periodic audit on the surgical safety checklist implementation. • Implement policy and procedure for incorrect count of instruments and sponges in the OT. • Ensure compliance. • Foster a culture of safety.

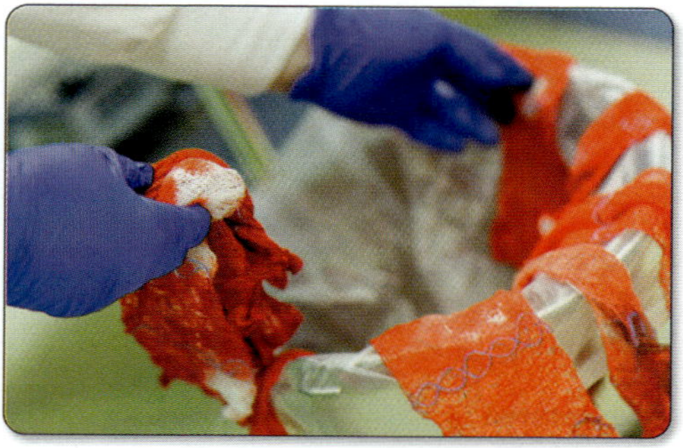

Figure 96 Counting of sponge in operation theater

Event-Based Learning Summary

The key takeaways from this incident are crystal clear—there is no room for bypassing safe practices in surgical procedures. Adhering diligently to the WHO surgical safety checklist is imperative. Any deviation from this checklist can result not only in prolonged anesthesia time, potential dissatisfaction from the surgeon despite a successful surgery but also pose a significant risk of legal consequences for the organization and the entire surgical team. This case underscores the critical importance of maintaining meticulous counts during surgical procedures and ensuring efficient communication among all surgical team members to prevent such errors.

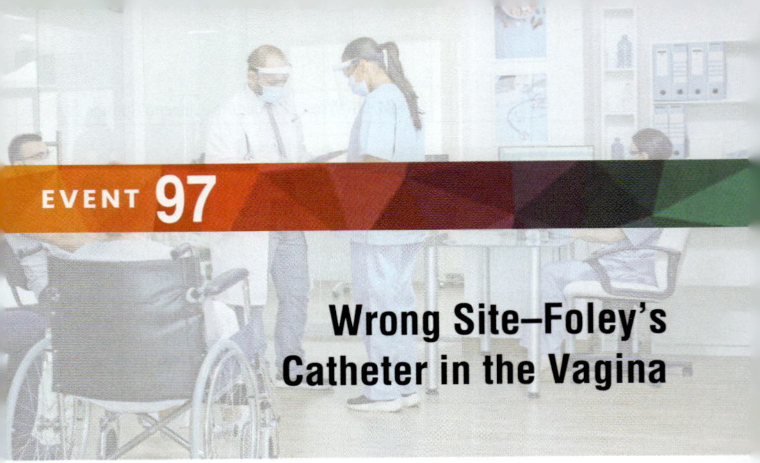

EVENT 97

Wrong Site–Foley's Catheter in the Vagina

EVENT NO.	PSE/097/092022
IPSG RELATED TO	IPSG 4 – Ensure Correct Site, Correct Procedure, Correct Patient Surgery

CASE STUDY DESCRIPTION

Ms Mona, a primi gravida with term pregnancy, got admitted for safe confinement. Since there was no progress in labour, the obstetrician decided to take her up for elective lower segment cesarean section (LSCS). The staff nurse did all the preoperative preparation and did Foley's catheterization in the ward. She ensured the urine flow in the kidney tray, advanced the catheter inside, secured it, and shifted the patient to OT. On the OT table, it was found that the Foley's catheter was inside the vagina rather than the urethral orifice, and the yellow-colored fluid which came out during catheterization in the ward was the leaked amniotic fluid, which was misinterpreted as urine. Foley's catheter was reinserted in OT. There was no untoward event that happened to the patient.

Positive Outcome

OT nurse rechecked the position of the catheter

Errors Encountered

- Foley's catheter was inserted into wrong site
- The staff failed to identify amniotic fluid and rather mistook it as urine.

Lessons Learned

For nurse	For nurse educator	For nurse administrator
• Use adequate lighting while performing the procedure. • Seek help for difficult procedures. • Do not perform procedures unless sure.	• To train all the nurses on the catheterization procedure with simulation. • Train nurses regarding potential difficult catheterization (obese, pregnancy, post delivery). • Observe live procedures.	• Annual competency check to be instituted for all the nurses. • Empower nurses to speak up when in doubt. • Privilege nurses for urinary catheterization.

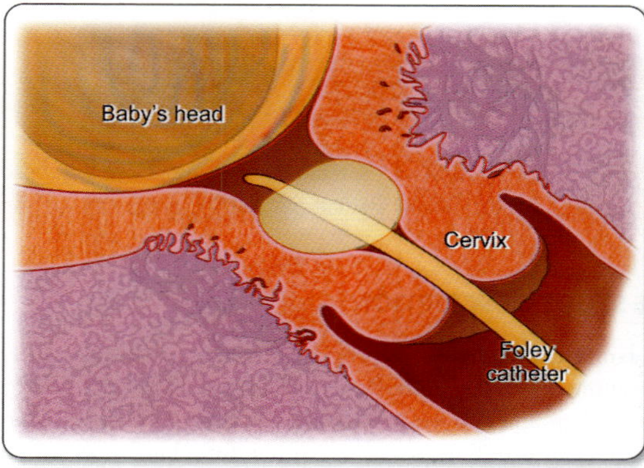

Figure 97 Insertion of urinary catheter into vagina

Event-Based Learning Summary

The critical takeaways from this incident emphasize the importance of precise patient preparation, especially in complex cases like Obstetric procedures. This event highlights the necessity for proper lighting, visualization, and positioning to identify anatomical structures correctly, particularly in gravid patients. It underscores the significance of effective communication within the healthcare team. The incident also led to a valuable policy revision for Obstetrics patient preparation in the ward. When in doubt, healthcare professionals must always express their concerns, fostering a culture of open communication to prevent such errors. Furthermore, thorough checks and verifications in the operating theater play a pivotal role in averting adverse events and ensuring patient safety. Current practice for LSCS is to catheterize in the OT under good lighting and is removed on the table after the LSCS.

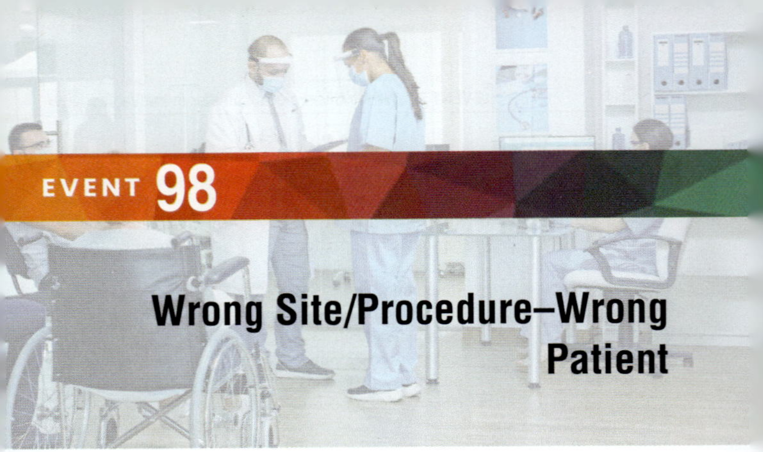

EVENT 98

Wrong Site/Procedure–Wrong Patient

EVENT NO.	PSE/098/092022
IPSG RELATED TO	IPSG 4 – Ensure Correct Site, Correct Procedure, Correct Patient Surgery

CASE STUDY DESCRIPTION

Mrs Laxmi Devi, a 64-year-old patient is suspected of bladder cancer and was awaiting her biopsy in the minor OT waiting room. She belonged to a rural background and was unaware of the procedure she was about to undergo. She was restless as she had to wait for a long time. After some time, the doctor in the OT called out Laxmi, and she was so glad that her turn came. She went to OT no. 2 for the procedure. The doctor and the team started the procedure of cystoscopy. The doctor was perplexed while doing the procedure as Laxmi's bladder seemed perfectly normal and showed no signs of cancer. After completing the procedure, the team asked for the patient's full name and details. To their surprise, they identified that they had performed the procedure on wrong patient. There was another patient named Laxmi Gayri, who was supposed to be taken for cystoscopy.

Positive Outcome

None.

Errors Encountered

- Wrong procedure was done.
- WHO surgical safety checklist was not utilized correctly.
- The patient was not involved in identifying herself and the procedure to be done.

Lessons Learned

For nurse	For nurse educator	For nurse administrator
• Patient identification with two sets of identifiers to be strictly adhered to. • Diligent practice of surgical safety checklist. • Involve patient in care. Questions must be asked to the patient as well.	• To train nurses on SSC and patient identification. • During training emphasize on involving patients to identify themselves and verify the procedure to be done.	• Conduct prevalence audits on process of identifying patient by involving them at the time of receiving the patient in the OT. • Ensure that the audit should be conducted by observing actual handover in the OT and also involving the patient. • Periodic audit on implementation of WHO surgical safety checklist must be implemented. • Audit findings must be discussed with the entire surgical team.

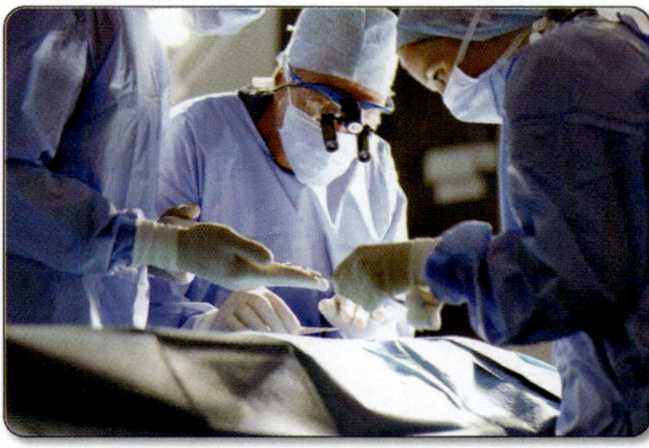

Figure 98 Cystoscopy procedure

Event-Based Learning Summary

This event underscores the critical importance of proper patient identification and effective communication in healthcare. Key takeaways from this incident include the necessity of patient education, ensuring patients are well-informed about their procedures, and practicing teach-back techniques to confirm their understanding. It also emphasizes the importance of diligently adhering to the WHO surgical safety checklist to prevent such errors.

Moreover, involving the patient directly in the confirmation of their name, procedure, and site is the most effective safety measure that healthcare providers can adopt. This direct engagement with the patient adds an extra layer of security to the identification process, reducing the risk of wrong-site or wrong-procedure errors. This approach empowers patients to actively participate in their care and provides an opportunity for them to raise any concerns or discrepancies, further enhancing overall patient safety.

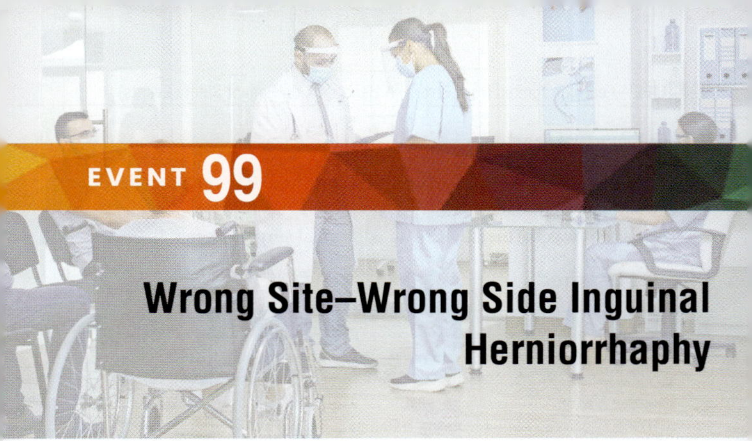

EVENT 99

Wrong Site–Wrong Side Inguinal Herniorrhaphy

EVENT NO.	PSE/099/092022
IPSG RELATED TO	IPSG 4 – Ensure Correct Site, Correct Procedure, Correct Patient Surgery

CASE STUDY DESCRIPTION

Mr Santosh was admitted to the surgical unit for left inguinal hernia repair. He was brought to the OT as the first patient for inguinal hernioplasty. The team prepped Mr Santosh and proceeded with the surgery. While on the table, the surgeon exclaimed that the hernia did not seem as big as he had examined. After the surgery, while removing the drapes, the scrub nurse noticed a huge swelling over the opposite inguinal region from the currently completed surgery and prompted the surgeons. The team realized that they had operated on the wrong side. They had operated on the left side instead of the right side. They again prepared the patient and operated on the right side.

Positive Outcome

None.

Errors Encountered

- The team did not perform the surgical sign-in and time-out procedures.
- The site was unmarked.
- The patient was harmed by having additional surgery done.

Lessons Learned

For nurse	For nurse educator	For nurse administrator
• Adherence to surgical safety checklist and site marking needs to be ensured. • Involve patients in care. Questions must be asked to patient as well. • OT nurses must ensure surgery is done only if the site is marked.	• Train nurses on surgical safety checklist. • During trainings emphasise on the importance of site marking. • Train nurses to speak up when surgical safety protocols are not followed. • Demonstrate surgical site verification.	• Conduct periodic audit on the surgical safety checklist implementation. • List of procedures requiring site marking to be developed. • Empower OT nurses to speak up and stop procedure if sign-in and Time-out policy are not followed. • Promote a culture of safety.

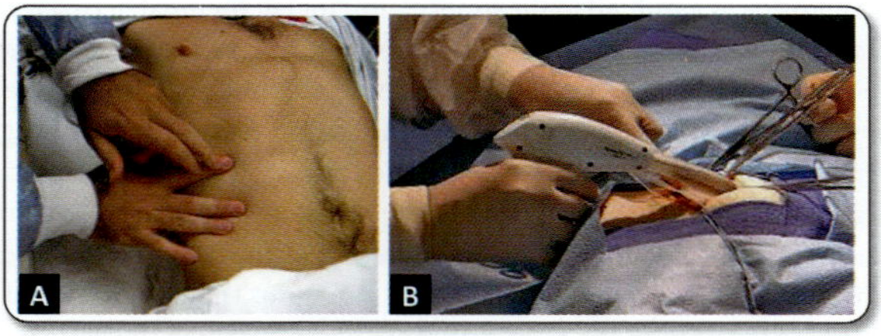

Figures 99A and B (A) An examination of hernia at right side; (B) Surgery of hernia at left side

Event-Based Learning Summary

This incident highlights the critical importance of adhering to surgical safety protocols, such as the surgical sign-in and time-out procedures. The absence of these safety measures, along with the failure to mark the surgical site, created a situation where the wrong side was operated on.

Key takeaways from this event include the need for healthcare teams to perform thorough surgical sign-in and time-out procedures from the beginning of the surgical process. Marking the surgical site before the operation is also crucial. These measures serve as critical safety checks to ensure that the correct procedure is performed on the correct site, ultimately preventing harm to the patient. In this case, prompt recognition of the error and corrective action helped prevent further complications, emphasizing the importance of immediate action when such incidents occur.

Involving the patient directly in confirming their identity, the planned surgery, and the intended surgical site adds an extra layer of protection to the surgical process. The patient, being the constant presence throughout their healthcare journey, can play a pivotal role in preventing wrong-site or wrong-procedure errors. This approach aligns with the principles of patient-centered care and empowers the patient to participate in their own safety actively. By asking the patient to state their name, the planned surgery, and the surgical site, the healthcare team can further mitigate the risk of incorrect procedures, ensuring patient safety and satisfaction.

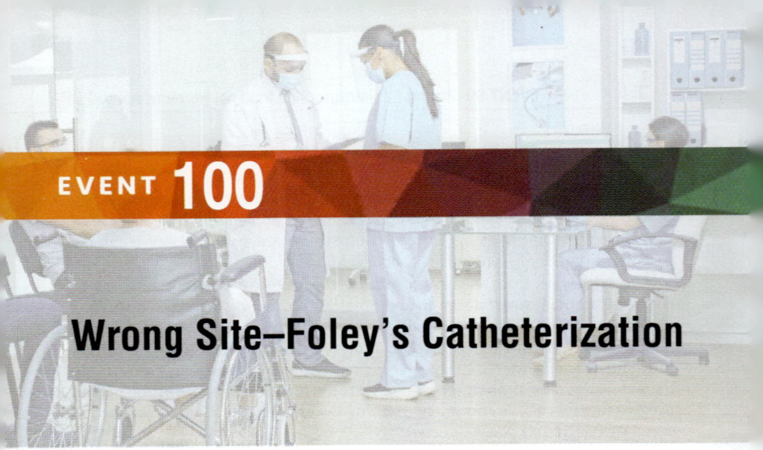

EVENT **100**

Wrong Site–Foley's Catheterization

EVENT NO.	PSE/100/092022
IPSG RELATED TO	IPSG 4 – Ensure Correct Site, Correct Procedure, Correct Patient Surgery

CASE STUDY DESCRIPTION

Ms Meenakshi, a 50-year-old female, complained of a lump in her right breast that persists through her menstrual cycle. She was diagnosed with Stages II (early-stage) right-side breast cancer and was admitted for partial mastectomy surgery. As per the preoperative orders, the staff nurse completed all the preoperative preparations, including Foley's catheterization in the ward. The OT in-charge checked as she saw the urine bag empty when receiving the patient into OT. Foley's catheter was reinserted in OT. In the OT, it was found that the Foley's catheter was in the vagina rather than in the urethra.

Positive Outcomes

- The OT In-charge had checked and found that the patient's urinary bag was not draining urine before receiving the patient from ward to OT.
- Timely identification prevented untoward issues for the patient.
- Catheterization was done before the surgery.

Errors Encountered

- The nurse was not diligent in inserting the catheter in the correct orifice.

- The foley's catheter was inserted in to the wrong orifice.
- The ward nurse failed to verify urine flow after the catheterization.

Lessons Learned

For nurse	For nurse educator	For nurse administrator
• Do not perform procedures unless sure. • Always verify urine flow after urinary catheterization • If there is no urine flow, inform to the senior or doctor immediately.	• Train nurses regarding potential difficult catheterization (obese, pregnancy, post delivery). • Observe live procedures.	• Annual competency check to be instituted for all the nurses. • Empower nurses to speak up when in doubt develop policies and procedures related to Foley's catheterization. • Privilege nurses for urinary catheterization.

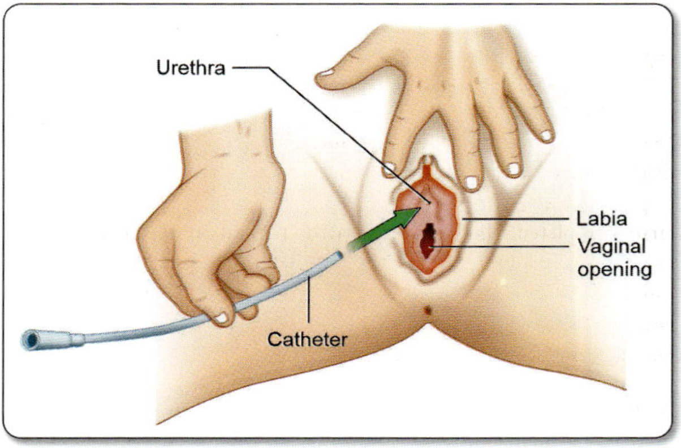

Figure 100 Right position of female catheterization

Event-Based Learning Summary

Wrong Site/Procedure events like the one described underscore the importance of diligent healthcare practices. Healthcare providers should always double-check and verify the correct placement of catheters and other medical devices. Adequate lighting, proper positioning, and clear communication are crucial in preventing such errors. If there is any doubt or uncertainty, it is vital for healthcare professionals to express their concerns and seek confirmation from their peers or supervisors. Diligence and thoroughness in every step of patient care are essential to ensure patient safety and prevent such unfortunate incidents. Proper verification procedures and adherence to protocols can go a long way in avoiding these errors.

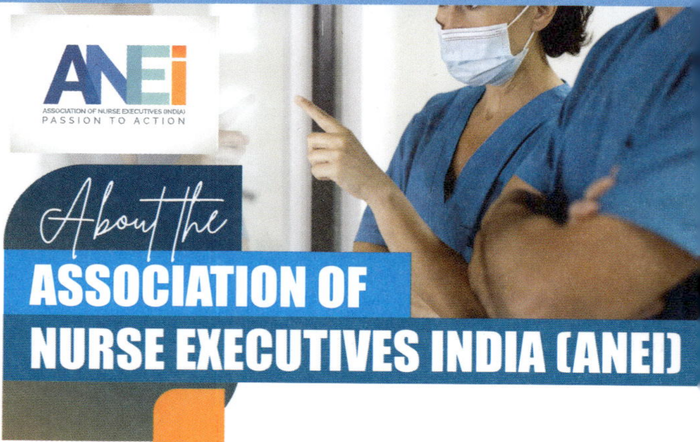

About the ASSOCIATION OF NURSE EXECUTIVES INDIA (ANEI)

The Association of Nurse Executives India (ANEI) is a dynamic professional body committed to the advancement of the nursing profession across India. Founded on the principles of leadership, professional development, and research; ANEI has been envisaged to play a pivotal role in shaping the future of nursing practice, education and research. By fostering collaboration among diverse stakeholders, including healthcare institutions, regulatory bodies, academic and professional organizations and other stakeholders, ANEI aims to elevate the standards of nursing and contribute to India's overarching health goals.

ANEI's vision is rooted in empowering nurses to be transformative leaders and advocates for safe and effective patient care. The organization serves as an inclusive platform, uniting voices from various domains of nursing—from education to practice. Through strategic partnerships and active engagement with policymakers, ANEI influences legislation, regulations, and reforms that directly impact the nursing profession. This ensures that nurses have a significant voice in shaping healthcare policies and practices.